Quiet BPD in Men

The Complete Guide to Recognizing, Understanding, and Healing from Internalized Borderline Personality Disorder

Ray Cabrera Mercado

Copyright © 2025 by Ray Cabrera Mercado. All rights reserved.

First Edition

ISBN: 978-1-7643271-4-5

This book is intended for educational and informational purposes only and is not intended to serve as medical advice. The information contained in this book is not intended to replace professional medical or psychological treatment, therapy, or counseling.

Readers should consult with qualified healthcare professionals before making any decisions related to their mental health, medical care, or treatment.

While the strategies and techniques described in this book are based on research and clinical observations, individual results may vary. The author makes no guarantees regarding the effectiveness of the information provided.

If you are experiencing thoughts of self-harm or suicide, please contact the National Suicide Prevention Lifeline at 988 or your local emergency services immediately.

All names, characters, case studies, and identifying details used in this book are fictional composites created for illustrative purposes. These composite characters represent common patterns and themes derived from research studies, clinical observations, anonymous surveys, and therapeutic consultations. No specific individual's story is represented. Any resemblance to actual persons, living or deceased, is purely coincidental.

Table of Contents

Preface 1

Chapter 1: The Successful Man's Secret Hell 5

Chapter 2: When Masculinity Becomes a Prison 16

Chapter 3: How Quiet BPD Develops in Men 26

Chapter 4: Decoding Your Quiet Chaos 38

Chapter 5: The Relationship Paradox 51

Chapter 6: Professional Success as Survival Strategy 64

Chapter 7: Getting the Right Help - Beyond Misdiagnosis 77

Chapter 8: Emotional Intelligence for the Logical Mind 85

Chapter 9: Building Connections That Heal 95

Chapter 10: Your Daily Recovery Arsenal 106

Chapter 11: For Partners, Families, and Allies 118

Chapter 12: From Surviving to Thriving - Your Future Self 132

References 146

Preface

Men don't typically pick up mental health books looking for academic dissertations or clinical jargon. We're story-driven creatures who understand concepts through examples, patterns, and real-world applications. We want to see ourselves in the narrative before we're willing to believe the science applies to us.

This book deliberately uses a story-first approach because research consistently shows that men are more likely to:

- Recognize themselves in narrative examples than in symptom checklists

- Engage with practical, action-oriented content over theoretical discussions

- Trust information that comes from someone who "gets it" rather than speaks about it academically

- Connect with authentic experiences rather than sanitized case studies

Throughout these pages, you'll encounter men like David, the executive who achieves everything but feels nothing. Marcus, who cycles through therapists who can't quite grasp what's happening beneath his successful exterior. Jake, who desperately wants connection but sabotages every relationship before it gets too close. Sarah's husband, who withdraws emotionally just when intimacy deepens.

These men, their stories, and all identifying details are fictional composites. They represent common themes, patterns, and experiences that have emerged from extensive research and clinical observation, including:

- Peer-reviewed studies examining male presentations of Borderline Personality Disorder
- Clinical observations from therapeutic work with men experiencing these symptoms
- Anonymous surveys and interviews with men who identified with Quiet BPD characteristics
- Support group discussions where men shared their experiences in confidential settings
- Conversations with partners and family members who witnessed these struggles
- Consultation with mental health professionals treating similar presentations
- Analysis of treatment outcomes and recovery patterns in male BPD populations

No single story represents any one individual. Instead, these composite characters embody the collective experiences of hundreds of men who have struggled with what we now understand as Quiet BPD. Their stories are designed to help you recognize patterns, understand possibilities, and see that recovery is not only possible but probable with the right approach.

How to Use This Book

This isn't a book you need to read cover to cover, though many men find that approach helpful. Each chapter builds on the previous ones, but you can also jump to sections that feel most relevant to your current situation.

If you're just beginning to suspect something is wrong: Start with Chapters 1-3 to understand recognition and development patterns.

If you're ready to take action: Focus on Chapters 7-10 for treatment and daily management strategies.

If you're supporting someone with these struggles: Chapter 11 is written specifically for partners, families, and allies.

If you're well into recovery: Chapter 12 addresses long-term thriving and giving back.

Each chapter includes practical tools, real-world applications, and actionable strategies. You'll find assessment questions, daily practices, communication scripts, and crisis management protocols. This book is designed to be a working manual, not just reading material.

A Note About Language and Approach

You won't find a lot of clinical terminology or therapeutic jargon in these pages. When technical terms are necessary, they're explained in straightforward language. The goal is understanding and application, not academic precision.

This book speaks directly to you as a man who may be struggling, not as a patient or a diagnosis. It acknowledges your intelligence, your capabilities, and your strength while addressing the very real pain you may be experiencing. It doesn't patronize or oversimplify, but it also doesn't hide behind professional distance.

The approach here is practical and solution-focused. While we'll explore the origins and patterns of Quiet BPD, the emphasis is always on what you can do about it. Every concept is connected to actionable steps you can take immediately.

What This Book Is Not

This book is not a substitute for professional treatment. It's a guide to understanding what you might be experiencing and a roadmap for getting the help that actually works. While the strategies and tools presented here are evidence-based and clinically sound, they work best when combined with appropriate professional support.

This book also doesn't promise quick fixes or miracle cures. Recovery from Quiet BPD is a process that typically unfolds over months and years, not days and weeks. What this book does promise is a clear understanding of what you're dealing with and proven strategies for managing it effectively.

Why This Matters Now

Male mental health is finally receiving the attention it deserves, but men with BPD have been largely overlooked in this conversation. The result is millions of men suffering in silence, cycling through ineffective treatments, destroying relationships they desperately want to save, and often turning to substances or other destructive behaviors to manage emotional pain they don't understand.

This book exists to change that pattern. It's the resource that should have been available years ago, written specifically for men who experience emotions intensely but have learned to hide that intensity behind walls of achievement, anger, or withdrawal.

Your struggle is real. Your pain matters. And recovery is not only possible—it's happening every day for men who finally understand what they're dealing with and how to address it effectively.

The journey from silent suffering to authentic strength begins with understanding. And understanding begins with recognizing yourself in these pages.

Welcome to a conversation that's long overdue.

Chapter 1: The Successful Man's Secret Hell

You've built the perfect life. So why does it feel like you're drowning?

Marcus sits in his corner office on the forty-second floor, staring out at the city skyline. The view that once filled him with pride now feels like a prison window. At thirty-eight, he's everything society says a man should be. Vice President of Operations. Six-figure salary. Beautiful wife. Two kids in private school. BMW in the driveway.

But here's what nobody sees: Marcus hasn't felt genuinely happy in years. He goes through the motions, performs his roles, and maintains the facade. Inside, though, there's nothing but a gnawing emptiness and a constant fear that everyone will discover he's a fraud.

Last week, his wife Sarah asked him why he never seems present anymore. "You're here, but you're not really here," she said. Marcus wanted to explain, but he couldn't find the words. How do you tell someone that you feel like you're suffocating in your own life? That success feels like quicksand? That you're terrified people will see through the performance?

This is the reality for millions of successful men living with what mental health professionals call **Quiet Borderline Personality Disorder**. Unlike the dramatic, outward chaos often associated with BPD, Quiet BPD turns all that emotional turmoil inward. You become your own prisoner, your own harshest critic, your own worst enemy.

The Quiet BPD Reality

Why Your Therapist Missed It

If you've sought help before, there's a good chance you walked away with the wrong diagnosis. Maybe you were told you have depression, anxiety, ADHD, or even bipolar disorder. Perhaps a therapist suggested you have "anger management issues" or recommended couples counseling for your relationship problems.

Here's why this happens so often with men: **diagnostic bias runs deep in mental health**. Most BPD research has focused on women, creating a blind spot when it comes to recognizing how this condition manifests in men. The diagnostic criteria were essentially built around female presentation patterns, missing the unique ways men experience and express emotional dysregulation.

Research shows that men with BPD are significantly more likely to be misdiagnosed with other conditions. We're seen as angry rather than scared, controlling rather than desperate for connection, and emotionally unavailable rather than emotionally overwhelmed. The very traits that society teaches us make us "good men" - stoicism, self-reliance, emotional control - become the mask that hides our suffering.

Mental health professionals often miss Quiet BPD in men because we've learned to internalize our chaos. We don't throw things or make dramatic scenes. Instead, we withdraw, work obsessively, drink too much, or simply go numb. Our distress signal looks like success from the outside.

The Imposter Behind the Achievement Mask

Maybe you recognize this pattern: You achieve something significant - a promotion, closing a big deal, buying the house you wanted - and instead of satisfaction, you feel... empty. Or worse, terrified that someone will figure out you don't deserve it.

This is the imposter syndrome that plagues many men with Quiet BPD. **Achievement becomes both our drug and our prison**. We chase external validation because our internal sense of self is so unstable. Each success provides a temporary high, a momentary relief from the gnawing question: "Who am I really?"

But here's the trap: the higher you climb, the further you have to fall. The more successful you become, the more you have to lose. The imposter feeling doesn't go away with achievement - it grows stronger. You start believing that your entire life is built on a lie that everyone else can see through.

Different from Classic BPD

You might be thinking, "But I'm not like those people with BPD I've heard about." You're right. Classic BPD - what researchers call "externalized" BPD - involves outward emotional explosions, dramatic relationship patterns, and behaviors that are hard to miss.

Quiet BPD is the opposite. Your emotional storms happen inside. Instead of lashing out at others, you attack yourself. Instead of dramatic breakups, you slowly withdraw from relationships. Instead of obvious self-destructive behaviors, you engage in socially acceptable forms of self-harm like overworking, perfectionism, or substance use.

The emotional intensity is just as real, but you've learned to contain it. You might experience:

- Intense inner criticism that you'd never voice to another person
- Emotional numbness that you mistake for being "logical" or "practical"
- Chronic feelings of emptiness despite external success
- Fear of abandonment that makes you push people away first
- Identity confusion masked as "being adaptable" or "going with the flow"
- Anger that you turn inward, leading to depression and self-punishment

The Male Mental Health Crisis Hiding in Plain Sight

The statistics are staggering and heartbreaking. Men are three times more likely to die by suicide than women. We're significantly less likely to seek mental health treatment. When we do seek help, we're more likely to drop out of therapy or receive inadequate treatment.

The problem isn't that men don't have mental health issues - it's that our issues often go unrecognized. We've been conditioned to suffer in silence, to view emotional struggles as personal failures rather than treatable conditions. The phrase "man up" has become emotional suicide instructions.

Men with BPD face additional challenges. The condition is still widely misunderstood as a "women's disorder," leading to delayed diagnosis, inappropriate treatment, and increased stigma. Many men spend years or even decades struggling with symptoms that have a name, a cause, and effective treatments.

Self-Recognition Section

The 20-Question Quiet BPD Assessment for Men

Answer honestly. There's no judgment here, only recognition:

1. Do you feel like you're performing the role of your life rather than living it?
2. Does success feel empty or temporary, leaving you wondering "What's next?"
3. Do you struggle with a sense of who you really are beneath your professional identity?
4. Do you fear that people would reject you if they knew the "real" you?
5. Do you find yourself withdrawing from relationships when they become too close?
6. Do you experience intense inner criticism that you'd never direct at another person?
7. Do you use work, substances, or other activities to avoid dealing with emotions?

8. Do you feel emotionally numb much of the time, even during significant events?
9. Do you have difficulty trusting your own perceptions and decisions?
10. Do you feel like you're walking on eggshells around your own emotions?
11. Do you struggle with chronic feelings of emptiness or meaninglessness?
12. Do you find yourself people-pleasing or agreeing to things you don't want to do?
13. Do you have intense reactions to criticism or perceived rejection?
14. Do you find it difficult to ask for help, even when you need it?
15. Do you experience mood swings that others don't see?
16. Do you feel like you have to be perfect to be acceptable?
17. Do you struggle with abandonment fears while simultaneously pushing people away?
18. Do you engage in self-sabotage when things are going well?
19. Do you have difficulty expressing needs or emotions in relationships?
20. Do you feel like you're living someone else's life rather than your own?

If you answered "yes" to more than half of these questions, you might be dealing with Quiet BPD. This isn't a clinical diagnosis - only a qualified mental health professional can provide that. But it might be the first step toward understanding why you feel the way you do.

Common Misdiagnoses You May Have Received

Many men with Quiet BPD have been down the diagnostic road before. You might have received one or more of these labels:

Depression: While depression often co-occurs with BPD, antidepressants alone rarely address the core identity and relationship issues of BPD.

Anxiety Disorders: The constant hypervigilance and fear of abandonment in BPD can look like generalized anxiety or social anxiety.

ADHD: The inner chaos and difficulty with focus can resemble attention deficit issues.

Bipolar Disorder: The mood instability in BPD is often mistaken for bipolar, but the patterns are different.

Anger Management Issues: The intense emotions of BPD, when they do surface, can be mislabeled as simple anger problems.

Narcissistic Personality Disorder: The defensive grandiosity that some men develop to cope with BPD can be mistaken for narcissism.

Why Traditional Therapy Hasn't Worked

If you've tried therapy before and felt like it didn't help, you're not alone. Many men with Quiet BPD have frustrating therapy experiences. Here's why:

Wrong Treatment Approach: If you were misdiagnosed, you likely received treatment designed for other conditions. Cognitive Behavioral Therapy (CBT) for depression works differently than therapy specifically designed for personality disorders.

Therapist Lack of Training: Not all therapists are trained to recognize or treat personality disorders, especially in men. Many graduate programs spend minimal time on BPD, and even less on male presentation.

Therapeutic Mismatch: Some therapy approaches require emotional openness that feels impossible when you're used to keeping everything inside. You might have felt pressured to "open up" before you felt safe doing so.

Male Communication Styles: Traditional talk therapy doesn't always match how men process and communicate emotions. You might have felt like you were speaking different languages.

Physical Symptoms You've Been Ignoring

Quiet BPD doesn't just affect your emotions - it shows up in your body too. You might have been attributing these symptoms to stress, aging, or other causes:

- Chronic fatigue despite adequate sleep
- Headaches or muscle tension, especially in the jaw, neck, and shoulders
- Digestive issues with no clear medical cause
- Sleep disturbances or insomnia
- Changes in appetite or eating patterns
- Increased susceptibility to illness
- Chest tightness or breathing difficulties during stress
- Physical restlessness or inability to sit still

These symptoms make sense when you understand that your body has been in a constant state of hypervigilance, trying to protect you from perceived threats to your emotional safety.

Hope and Framework

Recovery Stories from Men Who've Made It

Let me tell you about David, a successful attorney who came to understand his Quiet BPD at age forty-two. For years, he'd been the perfect lawyer, husband, and father on paper. Inside, he felt like a fraud waiting to be exposed. His marriage was distant, his relationship with his teenage kids was strained, and he was drinking more each year to cope with the emptiness.

Recovery wasn't easy, but it was possible. Today, David describes feeling "real" for the first time in his adult life. He's learned to recognize his emotions instead of numbing them, to communicate his needs instead of expecting people to read his mind, and to find his identity beyond his achievements. His marriage is stronger than ever, his kids actually seek him out for conversations, and he hasn't had a drink in over two years.

Then there's Michael, a tech executive who realized at thirty-five that his perfectionism and workaholism were actually symptoms of something deeper. Through specialized therapy and hard work, he learned that vulnerability wasn't weakness - it was the foundation of authentic connection. He's now in the healthiest relationship of his life and has found ways to channel his intensity into meaningful work and relationships.

These aren't isolated stories. Men with Quiet BPD can and do recover. The key is getting the right understanding, the right treatment, and the right support.

What This Journey Will Require

Recovery from Quiet BPD isn't about fixing what's broken - it's about understanding what's been adaptive and learning new ways to get your needs met. This journey will ask several things of you:

Courage to Feel: You'll need to gradually let yourself experience emotions you've been avoiding. This sounds simple, but for someone who's spent years in emotional shutdown, it can feel overwhelming at first.

Willingness to Be Seen: Recovery involves slowly dropping the masks and letting trusted people see who you really are. This is terrifying when you've believed your authentic self is unacceptable.

Patience with the Process: Personality patterns took years or decades to develop. Changing them takes time too. Progress isn't always linear, and setbacks don't mean failure.

Commitment to New Ways of Thinking: You'll need to challenge beliefs about yourself and relationships that feel like fundamental truths but are actually learned patterns from your past.

Investment in Relationships: Recovery happens in relationship with others. You'll need to gradually practice vulnerability, communication, and trust in safe relationships.

The Book's Promise

This book won't promise you a quick fix or a complete personality transformation. What it will do is give you a roadmap from silent suffering to authentic strength. You'll learn:

- How to recognize and understand your emotions instead of being overwhelmed by them
- Ways to communicate your needs and boundaries in relationships
- Strategies for managing the intense inner criticism that's been your constant companion
- Tools for building genuine self-worth that doesn't depend on external achievement
- Methods for creating authentic connections instead of performing relationships
- Techniques for finding meaning and identity beyond your professional success

Most importantly, you'll learn that recovery is possible. Thousands of men have walked this path before you. You don't have to stay trapped in the secret hell of looking successful while feeling empty inside.

The journey ahead isn't easy, but it's worth it. You deserve to feel real. You deserve authentic connections. You deserve to live your actual life instead of performing a role. And despite what that inner critic tells you, you're worth the effort it's going to take.

What Happens in the Next 24 Hours

Right now, you might be feeling a mix of recognition, relief, and maybe some fear. That's normal. You've just named something that might have been haunting you for years. Here's what you can do in the next day to start this journey:

Give Yourself Credit: Recognizing these patterns takes courage. Most people spend their entire lives avoiding this level of self-awareness.

Resist the Urge to Judge: Your brain might start criticizing you for having these issues or for not recognizing them sooner. Notice these thoughts, but don't engage with them.

Share with One Trusted Person: If you have someone in your life who feels safe, consider sharing what you've learned. You don't have to share everything, but breaking the isolation is powerful.

Start a Simple Journal: Begin tracking your emotions and triggers. Nothing fancy - just note what you're feeling and what might have triggered it.

Research Therapists: Look for mental health professionals who specifically mention experience with personality disorders or DBT (Dialectical Behavior Therapy) on their websites.

Practice Self-Compassion: Talk to yourself the way you'd talk to a good friend who was struggling. You didn't choose to develop these patterns, and recognizing them is the first step toward freedom.

The most important thing to remember is this: **you're not broken**. You're not fundamentally flawed. You're not doomed to live this way forever. You're a person who developed very understandable coping mechanisms for difficult circumstances, and those mechanisms have outlived their usefulness.

The secret hell you've been living in has an exit door. You've just found it.

Chapter 2: When Masculinity Becomes a Prison

The very strength that helped you survive is now killing you slowly.

At six years old, James scraped his knee badly on the playground. Blood was dripping down his shin, and tears were streaming down his face. His father's response was immediate and clear: "Big boys don't cry. Suck it up."

That moment planted a seed that would grow for the next three decades. James learned that emotions were dangerous territory for males. Pain was to be endured silently. Fear was to be hidden. Sadness was weakness. The only acceptable emotion for a man was a controlled, productive anger - and even that had to be carefully managed.

By thirty-six, James had mastered the art of emotional suppression. He was successful, respected, and appeared to have everything together. But inside, he felt like he was suffocating. The emotions he'd been taught to ignore hadn't disappeared - they'd gone underground, creating an internal pressure cooker that was always one degree away from exploding.

This is the masculine trap that millions of men find themselves in. **The very traits that society rewarded in us as boys become the prison walls that contain us as men.**

The Masculine Wound

How "Man Up" Becomes Emotional Suicide

The phrase "man up" might be the most dangerous two words in the English language for male mental health. It sounds like encouragement, like a call to strength and resilience. In reality, it's often a death sentence for emotional development.

Every time a boy hears "man up," he learns that his natural emotional responses are unacceptable. Sadness becomes shame. Fear becomes something to hide. Vulnerability becomes a target for ridicule. **The message is clear: to be masculine, you must disconnect from half of the human experience.**

Research consistently shows that men who rigidly adhere to traditional masculine norms have higher rates of depression, anxiety, substance abuse, and suicide. The very traits that are supposed to make us strong - emotional stoicism, self-reliance, avoiding help-seeking - become the factors that destroy our mental health.

For men with Quiet BPD, this cultural programming is particularly devastating. BPD involves intense emotional experiences and difficulty regulating emotions. When you combine this with a lifetime of learning that emotions are weakness, you get a perfect storm of internal suffering.

The Boy Who Learned Feelings Were Dangerous

Picture a typical scene from boyhood. A young boy is upset about something - maybe he's been excluded from a game, maybe he's worried about a test, maybe he's just overwhelmed by the big emotions that all children experience.

In many families, this boy learns quickly that emotional expression leads to consequences. He might be told he's being "dramatic" or "too sensitive." He might be ignored until he stops showing emotions. He might even be punished for crying or expressing fear.

The boy doesn't stop having emotions - he learns to hide them. He develops an internal filing system where feelings get buried, suppressed, or transformed into something more acceptable. Fear becomes anger. Sadness becomes numbness. Loneliness becomes independence.

This emotional burial system works for a while. It helps boys navigate a world that often punishes male emotional expression. But like any burial ground, what gets put underground doesn't stay buried forever.

Those emotions eventually surface, often in ways that feel out of control and frightening.

Why Anger Became Your Only Emotional Language

If you grew up male in most cultures, you learned that anger was the one emotion that was sort of acceptable. Not explosive, violent anger - that would get you in trouble too. But controlled, righteous anger? Competitive anger? Anger that motivated action? That was manly.

Anger became the Swiss Army knife of male emotional expression. Feeling hurt? Express it as anger. Feeling scared? Let it come out as anger. Feeling disappointed, lonely, or sad? Anger was the acceptable translation.

The problem is that anger is often what researchers call a "secondary emotion." It's usually covering something more vulnerable underneath. When anger becomes your only emotional language, you lose the ability to identify and express your actual feelings. This creates a cascade of problems in relationships and self-understanding.

Men with Quiet BPD often struggle with this particularly intensely. The emotions underlying BPD - abandonment fears, identity confusion, intense shame - are exactly the kinds of vulnerable feelings that boys learn to convert into anger. But because Quiet BPD turns emotions inward, even the anger gets suppressed, creating an internal emotional volcano that never gets to erupt.

The Cost of the "Strong Silent Type" Mythology

The "strong silent type" is a beloved masculine archetype in our culture. Think Clint Eastwood in Westerns, action heroes who never show weakness, business leaders who make tough decisions without apparent emotional impact. This mythology suggests that true strength means feeling less, needing less, saying less.

But here's what the mythology doesn't tell you: **the strong silent type is often dying inside**.

Real strength includes the ability to recognize, understand, and appropriately express emotions. It includes the capacity for vulnerability, connection, and asking for help when needed. The "strong silent type" often represents not strength, but emotional disability - an inability to access the full range of human experience.

For men with Quiet BPD, this mythology is particularly damaging. It reinforces the idea that their intense inner emotional life is a sign of weakness rather than a sign that they're human beings dealing with the aftereffects of trauma and invalidation.

Male-Specific Manifestations

Workaholism as Socially Acceptable Self-Harm

In a culture that values productivity and achievement, workaholism doesn't look like a mental health symptom. It looks like dedication, ambition, and success. **But for many men with Quiet BPD, workaholism is a form of socially acceptable self-harm**.

Work becomes a place to hide from emotions, relationships, and internal chaos. The structure, deadlines, and external validation provide temporary relief from the inner emptiness and confusion. But like any addiction, workaholism requires increasing doses to achieve the same effect.

You might recognize these patterns:

- Working long hours to avoid going home and facing relationship issues
- Taking on more responsibilities than you can handle to feel important
- Checking emails obsessively, even during family time or vacations
- Feeling guilty or anxious when you're not being productive
- Using work achievements to justify your existence and worth

- Becoming irritable or depressed when work is slow or when you're between jobs

The tragedy is that workaholism often makes the core issues of BPD worse. It increases isolation, prevents the development of genuine relationships, and reinforces the belief that your worth is based on what you do rather than who you are.

Substance Use as Emotional Anesthesia

Men are more likely than women to use substances to cope with mental health issues. For men with Quiet BPD, substances often serve as emotional anesthesia - a way to numb the intense inner experience that feels too overwhelming to face directly.

Alcohol becomes liquid courage for social situations and liquid numbness for overwhelming emotions. It might help you feel more connected to others temporarily, or it might provide blessed relief from the constant internal criticism and emotional chaos.

But substance use creates a vicious cycle with BPD symptoms. While it provides temporary relief, it ultimately makes emotional regulation more difficult. It interferes with sleep, increases depression and anxiety, and prevents the development of healthy coping skills.

The substances don't have to be illegal or even obviously problematic. Many men with Quiet BPD develop dependencies on:

- Alcohol (often wine or beer, consumed "responsibly" but regularly)
- Marijuana (used to "relax" or "unwind")
- Prescription medications (anxiety or sleep medications used beyond their intended purpose)
- Caffeine (used to manage energy and mood throughout the day)
- Nicotine (vaping, smoking, or tobacco products for stress relief)

Risk-Taking and Adrenaline Addiction

Some men with Quiet BPD are drawn to high-risk activities or adrenaline-inducing experiences. This isn't necessarily extreme sports or dangerous behaviors - it might be financial risks, career gambles, or relationship choices that create drama and intensity.

Risk-taking can serve several functions for men with BPD. It provides a temporary escape from emotional numbness, creates external drama that matches the internal chaos, and offers opportunities for either triumph or self-punishment.

You might notice patterns like:

- Making impulsive career changes or business decisions
- Engaging in financial speculation or gambling
- Pursuing affairs or relationships that create chaos
- Driving aggressively or engaging in road rage
- Participating in extreme sports or dangerous hobbies
- Creating conflict or drama when life feels too stable

Sexual Compulsivity and Validation Seeking

For some men with Quiet BPD, sexuality becomes a way to seek validation, feel connected, or experience intensity. This might manifest as compulsive use of pornography, serial relationships, affairs, or other sexual behaviors that provide temporary relief from emptiness or self-doubt.

Sex can temporarily fill the void that BPD creates, providing physical intimacy when emotional intimacy feels too scary, and offering validation when self-worth is unstable. But like other addictive behaviors, sexual compulsivity often increases shame and creates more problems than it solves.

Physical Aggression Turned Inward

While women with BPD might engage in self-harm behaviors like cutting, men often turn their aggression inward in different ways. This might include:

- Punching walls, doors, or other objects when frustrated
- Engaging in unnecessarily rough sports or physical activities
- Neglecting physical health through poor diet, sleep, or medical care
- Working out to the point of injury or exhaustion
- Engaging in physical labor or activities to exhaustion as self-punishment
- Hair pulling, nail biting, or other self-directed physical behaviors

These behaviors often feel like emotional release in the moment, but they reinforce the cycle of shame and self-hatred that drives BPD symptoms.

Redefining Masculine Strength

Emotional Courage as the Ultimate Masculinity

Real masculinity isn't about suppressing emotions - it's about having the courage to feel them, understand them, and respond to them appropriately. **The man who can acknowledge his fears is braver than the man who pretends not to have any**. The man who can express sadness without shame is stronger than the man who numbs all his feelings.

Emotional courage means:

- Admitting when you're struggling instead of pretending to have everything together
- Asking for help when you need it rather than suffering in isolation

- Setting boundaries in relationships instead of either people-pleasing or pushing everyone away
- Expressing vulnerability appropriately rather than either oversharing or sharing nothing
- Taking responsibility for your emotional impact on others
- Choosing conscious responses to emotions rather than reactive behaviors

This kind of emotional courage takes practice, especially if you've spent years learning to suppress feelings. But it's the foundation of genuine strength and authentic relationships.

Historical Warrior Cultures and Emotional Intelligence

Many traditional masculine archetypes actually included emotional intelligence as a crucial component of strength. Ancient warrior cultures often emphasized the importance of brotherhood, emotional bonds between fighters, and the ability to process trauma and loss together.

Greek warriors had deep friendships that included emotional intimacy. Native American warrior traditions included rituals for processing grief and trauma. Medieval codes of chivalry emphasized compassion, loyalty, and emotional honor alongside physical prowess.

The emotionally disconnected masculine ideal is actually a relatively recent historical development, largely arising from industrialization and the demands of modern warfare. Traditional masculine strength often included emotional depth, not emotional suppression.

Modern Male Role Models in Recovery

There are increasing numbers of men speaking openly about their mental health struggles and recovery journeys. Athletes, actors, business leaders, and everyday men are beginning to share their experiences with depression, anxiety, trauma, and personality disorders.

These men demonstrate that seeking help doesn't diminish masculinity - it enhances it. They show that emotional intelligence and vulnerability can coexist with strength, success, and respect. They prove that recovery is possible and that authentic masculinity includes the full range of human experience.

Permission to Feel Without Losing Your Identity

One of the biggest fears men face when beginning to address their emotional health is that they'll lose their masculine identity. There's a worry that feeling emotions means becoming weak, dependent, or somehow less male.

This fear is understandable but unfounded. Emotions are part of human experience, not gendered experience. Men who learn to feel and express emotions appropriately don't become less masculine - they become more fully human.

You can maintain your masculine identity while also:

- Acknowledging when you're hurt, scared, or sad
- Asking for support from friends, family, or professionals
- Expressing affection and care for people you love
- Admitting mistakes and making amends
- Setting boundaries based on your needs and values
- Choosing vulnerability in appropriate relationships

The goal isn't to become a different person. The goal is to become more authentically yourself - including the parts of yourself you've been taught to hide or suppress.

Moving Forward

The masculine prison you might find yourself in wasn't built in a day, and it won't be dismantled overnight. But every recognition of these patterns, every moment of choosing emotional honesty over suppression, every instance of reaching out instead of isolating is a small act of liberation.

The strength that helped you survive childhood, navigate school, build a career, and maintain relationships isn't weakness - it's evidence of your resilience and adaptability. **Now it's time to adapt again, this time toward authenticity rather than performance.**

The boy who learned to hide his feelings did what he needed to survive in his environment. The man you're becoming can learn new ways to thrive in relationships, in work, and in life. The prison of traditional masculinity has a door, and you're the one holding the key.

In the next chapter, we'll explore how these masculine patterns combined with other factors to create the perfect storm that led to your Quiet BPD. Understanding the origins of these patterns is the first step toward transforming them from limitations into strengths.

Remember: questioning these patterns doesn't make you less of a man. It makes you a man who's brave enough to choose growth over stagnation, authenticity over performance, and connection over isolation. That takes real courage.

Chapter 3: How Quiet BPD Develops in Men

Your symptoms aren't character flaws - they're survival strategies that no longer serve you.

Tommy was eight when his father came back from his second deployment. The man who returned wasn't the same person who had left. Dad was jumpy, distant, and angry. He'd sit in his chair for hours, staring at nothing. When Tommy tried to show him a drawing or share something about school, his father would either not respond at all or snap at him to "leave me alone."

Tommy learned to read the room, to stay quiet when Dad was having a bad day, to be the "good kid" who didn't cause problems. He learned that his needs weren't as important as keeping the peace. He learned that love was conditional on being invisible, helpful, and never too much trouble.

By the time Tommy reached adolescence, he was the perfect student, athlete, and son - on the outside. Inside, he felt empty, confused about who he really was, and terrified of being abandoned. He'd developed what would later be recognized as Quiet BPD, but at the time, everyone saw a successful, well-behaved young man who seemed to have it all together.

Tommy's story illustrates how Quiet BPD develops - not from one traumatic event, but from a thousand small moments that teach a child that his authentic self is unacceptable.

The Father Wound

Emotionally Unavailable Fathers and the Cycle of Silence

The relationship between a father and son creates a template for how that boy will relate to himself and others for the rest of his life. When that relationship is characterized by emotional unavailability, criticism, or neglect, it can create lasting wounds that contribute to the development of BPD.

Emotionally unavailable fathers come in many forms. There's the father who's physically absent due to work, divorce, or abandonment. There's the father who's physically present but emotionally checked out, going through the motions of parenting without real engagement. There's the father who shows love only through criticism or "teaching moments," believing that pointing out flaws is how you help someone improve.

For boys, fathers often serve as the primary model for masculinity and emotional regulation. When that model demonstrates that emotions should be suppressed, that needs should not be expressed, and that connection happens through shared activities rather than authentic communication, boys learn to relate to themselves in the same way.

The father wound in BPD development often involves:

- Learning that your emotions are too much, too intense, or inappropriate
- Receiving attention only when you achieve something or behave perfectly
- Being criticized for natural childhood behaviors like being loud, messy, or emotional
- Experiencing your father as unpredictable - sometimes available, sometimes rejecting
- Feeling responsible for your father's emotional state or problems
- Learning that conflict means complete rejection rather than temporary disagreement

Military Families and Intergenerational Trauma

Military families face unique challenges that can contribute to BPD development in children. The combination of frequent deployments, high stress, rigid hierarchies, and exposure to trauma creates an environment where emotional expression may be seen as weakness or liability.

Military culture, while serving important purposes, often reinforces many of the factors that contribute to BPD:

- Emotional suppression as a survival skill
- Black-and-white thinking (mission success or failure)
- Hypervigilance and constant alertness to danger
- Difficulty with intimacy and emotional vulnerability
- Identity primarily based on role and achievement rather than personal qualities

Children in military families often develop what researchers call "military child syndrome" - a pattern of being adaptable, self-reliant, and emotionally controlled. While these traits can be strengths, they can also prevent the development of emotional intelligence and authentic self-expression.

When parents have their own trauma from military service, they may unconsciously pass on survival strategies that were adaptive in combat but are problematic in civilian family life. The hypervigilance, emotional numbing, and interpersonal distrust that help soldiers survive war can create emotional distance and instability in family relationships.

The Absent Father Who Was Physically Present

Perhaps one of the most confusing father wounds comes from having a father who was physically present but emotionally absent. This father shows up to family events, provides financially, and may even be involved in activities like coaching or helping with homework. But when it comes to emotional connection, understanding, or genuine interest in his child's inner world, he's simply not available.

This type of father wound can be particularly damaging because it's so hard to identify. There's no obvious trauma, no clear abandonment, no dramatic conflict. Instead, there's a chronic sense that something is missing, that you're not really seen or understood by the man who's supposed to be your primary male role model.

Boys with this experience often struggle with:

- Feeling like they're performing relationships rather than experiencing genuine connection
- Difficulty identifying their own emotions and needs
- A sense that they're fundamentally boring or uninteresting
- Confusion about what authentic masculinity looks like
- Problems with intimacy in adult relationships
- Chronic feelings of emptiness or meaninglessness

Competition vs. Connection with Male Figures

In many traditional masculine environments, relationships between males are structured around competition rather than connection. Fathers may relate to sons through sports, academic achievement, or other competitive activities. While shared activities can be bonding, when competition becomes the primary mode of connection, it can create problems.

Boys learn that their worth is determined by their performance relative to others. They learn to see other males as competitors rather than potential sources of support. They learn that vulnerability is a weakness that others will exploit.

This competitive framework can prevent the development of genuine male friendships and mentoring relationships. Instead of learning to seek support from other men, boys learn to see them as threats or judges. This isolation continues into adulthood, where many men struggle to form meaningful friendships or seek help from other men.

Biological and Environmental Factors

Testosterone, Emotional Regulation, and the Male Brain

While culture and environment play huge roles in BPD development, biology also contributes. The male brain develops differently than the female brain, and these differences can influence how emotional regulation develops and how BPD symptoms manifest.

Testosterone affects emotional processing in several ways:

- It can increase impulsivity and risk-taking behaviors
- It influences the development of brain regions involved in emotional regulation
- It affects stress response systems and recovery from emotional activation
- It contributes to the tendency to express distress through aggression rather than other emotions

Boys with naturally high emotional sensitivity may find it particularly difficult to navigate a world that expects them to be emotionally controlled. The combination of biological emotional intensity with cultural pressure to suppress emotions can create the perfect conditions for developing maladaptive coping strategies.

Research has also shown that males may be more vulnerable to certain types of early trauma, particularly trauma that involves shame, humiliation, or attacks on their developing sense of masculine identity.

Epigenetic Transmission of Trauma

One of the most important recent discoveries in trauma research is that traumatic experiences can be passed down through generations via epigenetic changes - modifications in how genes are expressed rather than changes in the genes themselves.

This means that your father's or grandfather's traumatic experiences may have influenced your own emotional vulnerability. If your father experienced combat trauma, childhood abuse, or other significant stressors, these experiences may have changed how his genes were expressed in ways that were passed on to you.

This isn't destiny - epigenetic changes can be influenced by environment and experience. But it helps explain why some children seem more vulnerable to developing BPD symptoms even when their childhoods don't seem particularly traumatic.

Understanding epigenetic transmission can also reduce self-blame. Your emotional sensitivity and struggles aren't character flaws or personal failings - they may be inherited responses to trauma that helped previous generations survive but are less helpful in your current environment.

Childhood Invalidation in Masculine Contexts

Childhood invalidation - having your emotional experiences dismissed, minimized, or criticized - is a key factor in BPD development. For boys, this invalidation often happens in specifically masculine contexts.

Common forms of masculine invalidation include:

- Being told that crying or expressing sadness is "babyish" or "for girls"
- Having fears or anxieties dismissed as cowardice or weakness
- Being pushed to "toughen up" when experiencing normal childhood struggles
- Having interests or behaviors criticized as "too sensitive" or "not masculine enough"

- Being taught that asking for help is a sign of weakness
- Learning that anger is the only acceptable emotional expression for males

This invalidation teaches boys that their natural emotional responses are wrong or unacceptable. They learn to distrust their own perceptions and feelings. They develop a critical internal voice that sounds like all the external voices that told them their emotions were wrong.

When Achievement Becomes Your Only Worth

Many boys learn early that they're valued for what they do rather than who they are. Love and attention become contingent on performance - in school, sports, behavior, or other achievements. While some performance expectations can be motivating, when achievement becomes the only source of worth, it creates serious problems.

Boys who learn that their value depends on achievement often develop:

- Perfectionism that makes mistakes feel like existential threats
- Identity confusion when they're not actively achieving something
- Difficulty with intrinsic motivation - only able to function with external validation
- Imposter syndrome - feeling like their achievements don't reflect their "real" worth
- Chronic anxiety about maintaining their level of performance
- Depression when achievements don't provide the expected satisfaction

This achievement-based worth system sets boys up for the empty success that many men with Quiet BPD experience in adulthood. They reach their goals but find no lasting satisfaction because their identity is built on external validation rather than internal self-knowledge.

The Development Timeline

Early Signs in Boyhood Often Dismissed

The early signs of what will become Quiet BPD are often dismissed in boys as "just being sensitive" or "going through a phase." Unlike more obvious behavioral problems, these signs can be subtle and may even be seen as positive traits.

Early warning signs often include:

- Being unusually compliant and "easy" compared to other children
- Difficulty making decisions without excessive input from adults
- Intense reactions to criticism or perceived rejection
- Problems with friendships - either too clingy or too withdrawn
- Perfectionism in school or activities that goes beyond normal conscientiousness
- Difficulty identifying or expressing emotions beyond "fine" or "mad"
- Physical symptoms like stomachaches or headaches with no clear medical cause
- Excessive worry about family members or intense fear of abandonment

Because these behaviors often don't cause problems for adults - in fact, they might make a child easier to manage - they're frequently overlooked or even reinforced. The quiet, compliant child who doesn't cause trouble may be developing serious internal struggles that won't become apparent until much later.

Adolescent Coping Through Sports/Achievement

Adolescence is when many boys with developing BPD discover coping mechanisms that will carry them through young adulthood. Sports, academic achievement, artistic pursuits, or other structured activities provide several benefits:

- External structure that helps with emotional regulation
- Clear goals and feedback systems
- Social connection through shared activities
- Physical outlets for emotional intensity
- Sources of identity and self-worth
- Adult approval and recognition

While these activities can be genuinely beneficial, they can also become maladaptive coping mechanisms when they're used primarily to avoid dealing with emotions or to maintain a false sense of self.

The teenage athlete who defines himself entirely through his sport, the academic achiever who falls apart when he gets a B, or the musician who can't function when he's not performing may be using these activities to avoid developing genuine emotional regulation skills and authentic self-knowledge.

Young Adult Relationship Patterns

Young adulthood is when the relationship patterns characteristic of BPD often first become apparent. This is when many men first experience serious romantic relationships, and the fears of abandonment, identity confusion, and emotional intensity that characterize BPD begin to create obvious problems.

Common patterns include:

- Serial relationships that follow a pattern of idealization followed by devaluation
- Difficulty with commitment due to fears of both abandonment and engulfment
- Using relationships to define identity rather than bringing a stable sense of self to relationships
- Intense jealousy or possessiveness alternating with emotional withdrawal
- Difficulty with conflict resolution - either avoiding conflict entirely or escalating minor disagreements
- Sexual relationships that feel more intense than emotionally intimate relationships

Many men first seek therapy during this period, often at the suggestion of partners who recognize that something deeper than normal relationship problems is occurring. Unfortunately, without understanding of BPD, these early therapeutic interventions often focus on communication skills or anger management rather than addressing the underlying emotional dysregulation.

The Midlife Crisis That's Actually BPD

For many men with unrecognized Quiet BPD, midlife brings what appears to be a classic "midlife crisis" but is actually the emergence of long-suppressed BPD symptoms. After decades of using work, achievement, and performance to manage their internal chaos, many men find that these strategies stop working effectively.

Common triggers for midlife BPD emergence include:

- Career plateaus or setbacks that threaten identity based on achievement
- Children growing up and leaving home, removing a source of structure and purpose

- Physical changes of aging that challenge feelings of control and competence
- Health scares that force confrontation with mortality and vulnerability
- Relationship problems that can no longer be ignored or managed through avoidance
- Death of parents or other significant figures that trigger abandonment fears

What looks like a midlife crisis - sudden career changes, relationship upheaval, new risky behaviors - may actually be the emergence of BPD symptoms that were managed through external structure for decades. This is often when men finally receive accurate diagnosis and begin appropriate treatment.

Understanding Your Story

As you read through these patterns, you might recognize elements of your own story. Maybe you see your father in the descriptions of emotionally unavailable men. Maybe you recognize the achievement-focused childhood or the adolescent coping through structured activities.

It's important to remember that recognizing these patterns isn't about blaming your parents or your past. Your parents did the best they could with the tools they had, likely dealing with their own unrecognized trauma and mental health issues. The cultural contexts that shaped your childhood were passed down through generations of people trying to survive and provide for their families.

Understanding the origins of your BPD symptoms serves several important purposes:

- It helps reduce self-blame and shame about your struggles
- It provides a framework for understanding why certain situations trigger intense reactions

- It identifies specific areas where healing work might be most beneficial
- It helps you develop compassion for your past self and current struggles
- It provides hope by showing that these patterns developed in response to specific circumstances and can be changed with appropriate intervention

Your symptoms developed as adaptive responses to challenging circumstances. The boy who learned to suppress his emotions, seek worth through achievement, and avoid vulnerability was doing what he needed to do to survive in his environment. **The man you are now can learn new strategies that serve you better in your current life**.

The perfect storm that created your Quiet BPD is in the past. The healing work happens in the present. And your future can look very different from your past once you understand what you're working with and begin applying the right tools and strategies.

Chapter 4: Decoding Your Quiet Chaos

High-functioning on the outside, fragmenting on the inside.

Robert sits in his BMW after another successful board meeting, staring at his phone. The presentation went perfectly. The quarterly numbers exceeded expectations. Three colleagues complimented his leadership. His assistant already sent a follow-up email with action items for the team.

So why does he feel absolutely nothing?

The emptiness gnaws at him as he drives home to his suburban house. His wife will ask about his day, and he'll say "fine" because he doesn't know how else to describe the strange disconnection between his external success and his internal void. His teenage daughter will barely look up from her phone, which somehow feels like both relief and abandonment.

Tonight, like most nights, he'll have two glasses of wine - maybe three - and scroll through his phone until he falls asleep on the couch. Tomorrow he'll wake up exhausted despite adequate sleep, shower away the residual anxiety, and put on his professional mask for another day of high-functioning performance.

Robert's experience captures the essence of Quiet BPD: looking successful while feeling empty, appearing calm while battling internal chaos, maintaining relationships while feeling fundamentally disconnected.

The Quiet BPD Symptom Profile

Emotional Numbness with Breakthrough Rage

The emotional experience of Quiet BPD resembles living under emotional anesthesia most of the time, with occasional breakthrough moments of intense feeling that seem to come from nowhere. You might go weeks or months feeling relatively little, describing your mood as "fine" or "okay" when people ask. This isn't contentment - it's the absence of feeling.

But numbness isn't the absence of emotion - it's suppressed emotion under pressure. Like a dam holding back water, that emotional suppression creates tremendous internal pressure. Eventually, something breaks through, and when it does, the intensity can be overwhelming.

These breakthrough moments often involve anger because it's the one emotion that many men learned was somewhat acceptable. But the anger isn't really about the immediate trigger - it's about months of accumulated frustration, disappointment, fear, and sadness that had nowhere to go. A minor work setback becomes devastating. A partner's innocent comment triggers rage. A child's normal behavior provokes an explosion that surprises everyone, including you.

The pattern becomes: numbness, pressure building, explosion, shame about the explosion, return to numbness. Each cycle reinforces the belief that your emotions are dangerous and unpredictable, leading to even more suppression and, eventually, more intense breakthroughs.

The Executive Who Can't Stop Achieving

Achievement becomes both the solution to and the problem with Quiet BPD. External success provides temporary relief from the internal emptiness, creating a structure for identity when your internal sense of self feels chaotic or nonexistent.

You might recognize this pattern: each goal you reach provides a brief sense of satisfaction, followed quickly by the question "What's next?" The promotion you worked toward for months feels empty within weeks. The project you completed successfully feels meaningless as soon as it's done. **Success becomes a drug with diminishing returns**

- you need bigger and bigger achievements to get the same emotional payoff.

This creates what psychologists call the "hedonic treadmill" - constantly striving for the next thing that will make you feel complete, successful, or worthwhile. But because the problem isn't external circumstances, external achievements can never provide lasting satisfaction.

The executive who can't stop achieving often experiences:

- Inability to enjoy successes once they're reached
- Immediate anxiety about maintaining current levels of performance
- Identity confusion during vacations, weekends, or periods without clear goals
- Relationship problems because achievement takes precedence over connection
- Physical and emotional exhaustion from constant striving
- Depression when achievements don't provide the expected emotional payoff

Identity Confusion Behind Professional Success

One of the most challenging aspects of Quiet BPD is the profound confusion about who you actually are underneath your professional identity. You might be highly successful and competent at work while feeling like you have no idea who you are as a person.

This identity confusion stems from years of getting validation for performance rather than for being yourself. You learned early that love, attention, and approval came when you did things right, achieved goals, or met expectations. You never learned what you actually liked, wanted, or valued independent of external approval.

Common experiences include:

- Feeling like you're playing a role rather than living authentically
- Difficulty making decisions about personal matters (unlike professional decisions, which feel clear)
- Not knowing what you enjoy when you're not working toward something
- Feeling like people don't really know the "real" you - and wondering if there is a real you
- Changing your personality depending on who you're with
- Feeling like an imposter even in areas where you're genuinely competent

This identity confusion becomes particularly problematic in close relationships, where authenticity and consistency are important. Partners may comment that you seem like "different people" in different situations, or that they feel like they don't really know you despite years together.

Chronic Emptiness Despite External Fulfillment

The experience of chronic emptiness is one of the most difficult BPD symptoms to explain to others. It's not sadness, which has content and usually relates to specific circumstances. It's not depression, which typically involves negative thoughts and feelings. **Emptiness is the absence of feeling, meaning, or connection - like being a well-functioning robot going through the motions of a human life**.

This emptiness persists regardless of external circumstances. You can feel empty while closing a major deal, celebrating a birthday, or even during positive family moments. The emptiness isn't situational - it's existential. It raises questions like "What's the point?" and "Is this all there is?" that can't be answered by changing circumstances.

Many men with Quiet BPD describe feeling like they're watching their lives from the outside, like they're living someone else's life, or like they're waiting for their "real" life to start. The emptiness creates a constant search for something - anything - that will provide meaning, purpose, or genuine feeling.

Internalized Self-Destruction Patterns

While classic BPD often involves outward self-destructive behaviors, Quiet BPD turns that destruction inward. Instead of cutting or dramatic suicide attempts, you engage in subtler forms of self-harm that look like personal choice or even admirable dedication.

Internalized self-destruction might include:

- Perfectionism that makes you miserable but looks like high standards
- Workaholism that damages your health and relationships but appears successful
- Self-isolation during difficult times when you most need support
- Harsh self-criticism that you'd never direct at another person
- Sabotaging good opportunities because you don't believe you deserve them
- Staying in situations that make you unhappy because you believe it's what you deserve
- Physical self-neglect disguised as being "low maintenance"

These patterns are often invisible to others and even to yourself because they're woven into behaviors that society rewards. The workaholic gets promoted. The perfectionist gets praised. The self-reliant man is seen as strong. But underneath, these patterns serve the same function as more obvious self-harm - they provide a way to punish yourself for being "fundamentally flawed."

Daily Life Impact Analysis

Morning: The Dread of Another Performance

Many men with Quiet BPD describe mornings as the worst part of their day. You might wake up with a sense of dread about facing another day of performing competence, connection, and contentment that you don't actually feel.

The morning routine becomes a process of putting on armor for the day. Shower away the anxiety. Choose clothes that project the right image. Check emails to see what performance will be required today. Drink coffee to generate the energy for another day of masking.

The dread isn't about specific tasks or challenges - it's about the exhaustion of maintaining a facade for another 12-16 hours. You know that you'll spend the day managing other people's perceptions, meeting expectations, and suppressing any authentic emotional responses that might leak through.

Some mornings, the mask feels impossibly heavy. You might sit in your car for extra minutes before going into the office, or spend longer in the bathroom just to have a few moments where you don't have to perform for anyone.

Workplace: Exhaustion from Constant Masking

Work often provides structure and distraction that make Quiet BPD symptoms more manageable, but it also requires constant emotional labor to maintain your professional persona. You become expert at reading rooms, managing others' emotions, and presenting exactly the right version of yourself for each situation.

This constant masking is exhausting in ways that are hard to explain to others. It's not just the work itself - it's the energy required to monitor and control your emotional expressions, voice tone, body language, and reactions throughout the day.

You might experience:

- Feeling drained after meetings that seemed routine to others

- Needing recovery time after social interactions at work
- Difficulty concentrating when emotions threaten to break through
- Physical tension from controlling your emotional expression
- Relief when working alone versus anxiety about isolation
- Perfectionist tendencies that slow down your actual productivity

The workplace becomes both a sanctuary (providing structure and identity) and a prison (requiring constant performance). You excel professionally while feeling increasingly disconnected from your authentic self.

Evening: Numbing Behaviors and Isolation

Evenings often bring a crash after a day of high-functioning performance. The mask comes off, but instead of relief, you might experience emptiness, anxiety, or emotional overwhelm that you've been suppressing all day.

This is when numbing behaviors typically emerge. Alcohol becomes a way to transition from "work mode" to "home mode." Television provides mindless distraction from internal chaos. Social media offers brief hits of connection without real vulnerability. Gaming, shopping, or other activities provide temporary escape from the exhaustion of being yourself.

But numbing behaviors create their own problems. They prevent you from processing the day's emotions, developing genuine relaxation skills, or connecting authentically with family members. They also often increase shame and self-criticism, feeding the cycle of internal destruction.

The evening routine might look like: arrive home, minimal interaction with family, engage in numbing activity until sleep, repeat. Partners and children learn not to expect genuine emotional availability during these times.

Relationships: Present but Not Connected

One of the most painful aspects of Quiet BPD is feeling disconnected even in your closest relationships. You might be physically present - attending family dinners, watching movies together, participating in conversations - but feel emotionally absent or removed.

This disconnection isn't intentional or mean-spirited - it's protective. Genuine emotional connection requires vulnerability, and vulnerability feels dangerous when your emotional world feels chaotic and unpredictable. It's safer to engage on a surface level than to risk exposing your authentic self and facing potential rejection.

Family members often describe you as:

- "Here but not here" during family activities
- Difficult to read emotionally
- Reliable for practical support but unavailable for emotional support
- Someone who "doesn't open up" or share feelings
- Present for activities but absent for deeper connection

This creates a particular loneliness - being surrounded by people who care about you while feeling fundamentally alone and unknown.

Weekends: Lost Without Work Structure

Weekends and vacations can be particularly challenging for men with Quiet BPD who rely on work structure to manage their internal chaos. Without clear external demands and expectations, the emptiness and emotional volatility become more apparent.

You might find yourself feeling more anxious, depressed, or irritable during periods that are supposed to be relaxing. The lack of structure removes one of your primary coping mechanisms, and suddenly you're faced with unstructured time and the potential for emotional experiences you usually avoid.

Common weekend experiences include:

- Difficulty deciding how to spend free time
- Creating work-like projects to provide structure
- Feeling guilty for not being productive
- Increased substance use or other numbing behaviors
- Conflict with family members who expect more emotional availability
- Relief when Monday arrives and structure returns

Tracking Your Patterns

Trigger Identification System

Understanding your specific triggers is crucial for managing Quiet BPD symptoms. But identifying triggers requires paying attention to subtle internal experiences rather than obvious external events.

Effective trigger tracking looks at four levels:

Environmental triggers: Specific places, people, or situations that consistently create emotional reactions. This might include performance reviews, social gatherings, family visits, or certain work environments.

Interpersonal triggers: Relationship patterns that activate your BPD symptoms. Common triggers include perceived criticism, feeling ignored or excluded, changes in relationship dynamics, or conflicts with authority figures.

Internal triggers: Thoughts, memories, or internal states that trigger emotional dysregulation. This might include perfectionist thoughts, memories of past failures, or physical sensations like fatigue or hunger.

Temporal triggers: Times of day, week, or year when you consistently struggle more. Many people notice patterns around anniversaries, holidays, work cycles, or even daily rhythms.

Effective trigger identification involves tracking not just what happened, but what you were thinking and feeling before the triggering event, during it, and afterward.

Emotional Intensity Scale (0-10)

Many men with Quiet BPD have difficulty identifying and rating their emotions because they've learned to suppress or ignore them. An emotional intensity scale helps develop emotional awareness by providing a concrete way to measure internal experiences.

A practical 0-10 scale might look like:

- 0-2: Emotional numbness, feeling "fine" or disconnected
- 3-4: Mild emotions that don't interfere with functioning
- 5-6: Moderate emotions that you notice but can manage
- 7-8: Strong emotions that affect your behavior and decision-making
- 9-10: Overwhelming emotions that feel out of control

The goal isn't to stay at a 5 all the time - that's not realistic or healthy. The goal is to develop awareness of your emotional states and patterns, and to recognize when you need to use coping strategies.

Behavioral Pattern Mapping

Tracking behavioral patterns helps identify the connections between your emotional states, triggers, and actions. This creates awareness of cycles that might otherwise feel random or uncontrollable.

Common behavioral patterns to track include:

Withdrawal patterns: When and how you isolate from others, what triggers withdrawal, and what helps you reconnect.

Achievement patterns: How you use work or accomplishments to manage emotions, when this becomes problematic, and what happens when achievements don't provide the expected relief.

Numbing patterns: What substances or activities you use to avoid emotions, when this becomes problematic, and what needs these behaviors are trying to meet.

Relationship patterns: How you respond to conflict, closeness, or perceived rejection, and what happens in your relationships during different emotional states.

Physical Symptom Checklist

Quiet BPD often manifests in physical symptoms that might seem unrelated to mental health. Tracking these symptoms helps you recognize the connection between your emotional and physical experiences.

Common physical symptoms include:

- Sleep disturbances (insomnia, nightmares, or excessive sleep)
- Digestive issues (nausea, stomach pain, or changes in appetite)
- Muscle tension (especially in jaw, neck, shoulders, or back)
- Headaches or migraines
- Fatigue despite adequate rest
- Changes in immune function (getting sick more often)
- Physical restlessness or inability to sit still

Relationship Impact Assessment

Understanding how your Quiet BPD symptoms affect your relationships helps motivate change and provides concrete goals for improvement. This assessment looks at different types of relationships and specific impacts.

Key relationships to assess:

Romantic partnership: How do your symptoms affect intimacy, communication, conflict resolution, and daily interactions?

Parenting: How does emotional numbing or volatility affect your connection with children and your ability to meet their emotional needs?

Friendships: What prevents deeper male friendships, and how does your emotional unavailability affect social connections?

Professional relationships: How does masking affect your workplace relationships, and what happens when the mask slips?

Extended family: How do family gatherings or interactions with parents/siblings trigger your symptoms?

Making Sense of Your Patterns

As you begin tracking these various aspects of your experience, patterns will emerge that help explain behaviors and reactions that might have seemed random or confusing. You might notice that your worst days follow certain types of interactions, that your numbness increases during specific seasons, or that your relationship conflicts follow predictable patterns.

This awareness is the first step toward change. You can't modify patterns you don't recognize, and you can't develop effective coping strategies without understanding what you're actually dealing with.

The goal of tracking isn't to judge your patterns or immediately change everything. It's to develop what psychologists call "wise mind" - the ability to observe your experiences with curiosity rather than criticism, and to use that information to make conscious choices rather than operating on autopilot.

Many men find that simply tracking their patterns for a few weeks creates significant changes in their experience. When you're paying attention to your emotional states, triggers, and behaviors, you automatically become more conscious and less reactive. You start catching yourself before falling into old patterns, and you begin seeing options where you previously saw only automatic responses.

The quiet chaos of Quiet BPD becomes less chaotic when you understand its patterns. **Your symptoms aren't random or meaningless - they're your psyche's attempt to manage overwhelming internal experiences with the tools you learned in childhood**. As you develop better tools and deeper understanding, the chaos becomes more manageable, and the quiet becomes less necessary.

The high-functioning facade isn't who you really are - it's a survival strategy that served you well but has outlived its usefulness. Underneath that facade is a person capable of genuine emotion, authentic connection, and sustainable success that doesn't require constant performance.

Chapter 5: The Relationship Paradox

You destroy the very connections you desperately need.

David met Sarah at a work conference three years ago. The connection was instant and intense - they talked until 3 AM about everything from childhood dreams to philosophical questions about the meaning of life. For the first time in his adult life, David felt truly seen and understood. Sarah was beautiful, intelligent, and seemed genuinely interested in who he was beneath his professional success.

But as their relationship deepened, something shifted. David found himself pulling back, creating distance through work travel, emotional withdrawal, and subtle criticism. When Sarah tried to get closer, he felt suffocated. When she gave him space, he felt abandoned. He began testing her commitment in small ways - showing up late, "forgetting" important dates, making comments about other women to see if she'd get jealous.

Sarah's confusion was evident. "I don't understand," she told him during one of their increasingly frequent arguments. "When we met, you couldn't get enough of me. Now it feels like you're looking for reasons to leave."

David's experience captures the central paradox of BPD relationships: desperately craving the very intimacy that feels terrifying and suffocating.

The Push-Pull Dynamic

Fearful-Avoidant Attachment Explained

The relationship patterns in Quiet BPD stem from what attachment researchers call "fearful-avoidant attachment" - also known as disorganized attachment. This pattern develops when children experience caregivers as both sources of comfort and sources of fear or pain.

For boys who develop this pattern, intimate relationships become impossible puzzles: the people who can provide love and safety are also the people who can hurt you most deeply. This creates an approach-avoidance conflict where you simultaneously move toward and away from the people you care about most.

In fearful-avoidant attachment, you experience:

- Intense desire for close relationships combined with fear of being hurt
- Difficulty trusting others while desperately wanting to trust someone
- Feeling suffocated when relationships get close but abandoned when partners need space
- Alternating between idealization and devaluation of the same person
- Self-sabotaging behaviors when relationships feel "too good to be true"
- Hypervigilance for signs of rejection while also creating conditions that might cause rejection

This attachment style explains why many men with Quiet BPD have a history of relationships that start intensely and end badly, often following similar patterns despite involving different partners.

Why You Test the People Who Love You

Testing behaviors in relationships serve a specific psychological function for people with BPD: they provide information about whether someone will stay despite your perceived flaws, and they offer a sense of control over the timing and nature of potential abandonment.

Common testing behaviors include:

Emotional tests: Sharing increasingly personal or difficult information to see if the partner will stay interested and supportive.

Loyalty tests: Creating situations where the partner must choose between you and other people or activities to prove their commitment.

Patience tests: Engaging in behaviors that would reasonably frustrate most people to see if this person will stick around.

Conflict tests: Starting arguments or creating drama to see how the partner responds to your anger or distress.

Availability tests: Making demands on the partner's time or attention to ensure they prioritize the relationship.

The paradox is that testing behaviors often create the very abandonment they're designed to prevent. Partners become exhausted by constant tests and eventually leave, which "confirms" your belief that people always abandon you eventually.

Creating Distance to Avoid Abandonment

One of the most confusing aspects of BPD relationship patterns is the tendency to create distance from partners as a way to avoid the pain of abandonment. This seems counterintuitive, but it serves important psychological functions.

Distance-creating behaviors include:

- Emotional withdrawal during times when connection would be most healing
- Starting arguments when things are going well to create familiar conflict
- Focusing intensely on work or other activities when partners want closeness

- Criticizing partners for traits you initially found attractive
- Developing crushes on other people when your primary relationship is stable
- Sabotaging special occasions or meaningful moments

This distance serves as emotional insurance. If you push people away first, you maintain some control over the abandonment process. It hurts less to be rejected when you were already pulling back than to be caught off guard by someone leaving when you felt completely open and vulnerable.

The Partner as Both Savior and Threat

In BPD relationships, partners often get cast in contradictory roles that reflect your internal conflict about intimacy and dependence. The same person who represents salvation from your emptiness and loneliness also represents the ultimate threat to your emotional safety.

Your partner becomes a savior when they:

- Provide relief from chronic emptiness through their attention and love
- Offer validation and worth that you can't provide for yourself
- Create structure and meaning in your life through the relationship
- Serve as proof that you're worthy of love despite your internal self-criticism

Your partner becomes a threat when they:

- Have the power to hurt you more deeply than anyone else
- Represent dependence that conflicts with your need for self-reliance
- Know your authentic self, including the parts you believe are unacceptable

- Could potentially abandon you and destroy the identity you've built around the relationship

This dual role creates impossible expectations for partners. They're expected to be consistently available and understanding while also maintaining their own lives and needs. They're supposed to love you unconditionally while accepting that you may push them away when that love feels overwhelming.

Male-Specific Relationship Patterns

Emotional Withdrawal vs. Explosive Anger

Men with Quiet BPD often manage relationship conflicts through two primary strategies: withdrawal and anger. These patterns reflect both BPD symptoms and masculine socialization about emotional expression.

Emotional withdrawal patterns include:

- Going silent during conflicts rather than expressing vulnerable emotions
- Physically removing yourself from emotional conversations
- Responding to relationship problems by working more or staying busy
- Using substances or activities to avoid dealing with relationship issues
- Giving brief, noncommittal responses when partners try to discuss problems
- Postponing difficult conversations indefinitely

Explosive anger patterns include:

- Intense rage reactions that seem disproportionate to the triggering event
- Anger that covers hurt, fear, or abandonment panic

- Using anger to create distance when intimacy feels overwhelming
- Explosive reactions followed by shame and withdrawal
- Difficulty repairing relationships after angry outbursts

Both patterns serve the same function: they prevent the vulnerability required for genuine emotional intimacy while expressing the intense emotions characteristic of BPD.

Using Work/Hobbies to Create Distance

For many men with Quiet BPD, work and hobbies become ways to regulate closeness in relationships. When intimacy feels overwhelming, you can always retreat into activities that provide legitimate reasons for being unavailable.

Work becomes a relationship regulator when you:

- Take on extra projects during times of relationship stress
- Travel for business more than necessary to create physical distance
- Work late to avoid coming home to emotional conversations
- Check emails during family time to maintain psychological distance
- Use work stress as a reason to be emotionally unavailable
- Schedule work activities during important personal events

Hobbies serve similar functions when they:

- Require significant time away from home and family
- Provide social connections that don't require emotional vulnerability
- Create legitimate reasons to avoid relationship responsibilities

- Offer achievement and identity outside the relationship
- Serve as escape from emotional intensity

The tragedy is that these activities, which could enrich your life and relationships, become barriers to the intimacy you actually crave.

Sexual Intensity as Intimacy Avoidance

For some men with Quiet BPD, sexual connection becomes a substitute for emotional intimacy. Sex provides physical closeness and intensity without requiring the vulnerability of emotional sharing.

This pattern might include:

- Having intense sexual relationships with limited emotional connection
- Using sex to reconnect after conflicts without addressing underlying issues
- Feeling more comfortable expressing yourself sexually than emotionally
- Pursuing sexual variety or novelty when emotional intimacy feels stagnant
- Using sexual performance to prove your worth as a partner
- Avoiding conversations about the relationship by initiating physical intimacy

While sexual connection can be an important part of intimate relationships, when it becomes the primary or only way you connect with partners, it prevents the development of emotional intimacy and understanding.

Control Through Caretaking

Many men with Quiet BPD attempt to control their fear of abandonment by becoming indispensable through caretaking behaviors. If you can make yourself essential to your partner's well-being or happiness, they're less likely to leave.

Caretaking control patterns include:

- Taking responsibility for your partner's emotions and problems
- Providing solutions for issues your partner could handle independently
- Making yourself financially indispensable through excessive generosity
- Managing household responsibilities to prove your value
- Anticipating and meeting your partner's needs before they express them
- Becoming hurt or angry when your caretaking efforts aren't appreciated

This pattern creates resentment on both sides. You become exhausted from over-functioning while feeling unappreciated. Your partner feels controlled and loses opportunities to develop independence and confidence.

Silent Treatment and Shutdown Cycles

The silent treatment is a common pattern in men with Quiet BPD, often alternating with periods of normal or even intense connection. These shutdown cycles reflect both your fear of emotional overwhelm and your difficulty expressing needs directly.

Shutdown cycles typically follow this pattern:

1. Building emotional intensity or relationship stress
2. Feeling overwhelmed by emotions you can't identify or express
3. Complete emotional withdrawal and minimal communication

4. Partner confusion, frustration, or attempts to reconnect
5. Eventually emerging from shutdown, often without discussing what happened
6. Period of reconnection or normalcy until stress builds again

This pattern is particularly damaging because it prevents resolution of underlying issues while creating insecurity and confusion for partners who don't understand what triggered the shutdown or how long it will last.

Impact Across Relationships

Romantic Partnerships: The Impossible Dance

Romantic relationships bear the brunt of BPD symptoms because they activate both your deepest needs and your greatest fears. The intensity of romantic love triggers both the craving for merger and the terror of being truly known.

Common patterns in romantic relationships include:

The idealization phase: New relationships feel perfect because they provide hope for finally being understood and loved unconditionally. You may move quickly toward commitment, share intensely personal information, and feel like you've found your soulmate.

The devaluation phase: As the relationship becomes more real and less idealized, flaws in your partner become magnified. You begin to doubt whether this person can really meet your needs or whether they truly understand you.

The testing phase: You begin behaviors designed to test your partner's commitment while simultaneously pushing them away to avoid the vulnerability of complete dependence.

The crisis phase: Conflicts become existential threats. Arguments feel like the end of the relationship. Your partner's normal needs for space or independence feel like abandonment.

The repair or ending phase: Either you develop skills to break these cycles and create more stable connection, or the relationship ends, often confirming your beliefs about being unlovable or relationships being impossible.

Fatherhood: Loving but Absent

Becoming a father creates unique challenges for men with Quiet BPD. Children need consistent emotional availability, but your symptoms make this difficult to provide. The result is often a pattern of loving but being emotionally absent or unpredictable.

Common fatherhood patterns include:

- Difficulty with the emotional demands of infants and young children
- Providing well financially while struggling with emotional provision
- Feeling overwhelmed by children's big emotions and normal developmental needs
- Either over-functioning (trying to be the perfect father) or under-functioning (withdrawing from parenting responsibilities)
- Difficulty with discipline that requires both firmness and emotional connection
- Fear of repeating patterns from your own childhood while lacking models for different approaches

Children often experience fathers with Quiet BPD as loving but unpredictable, present but emotionally distant, or caring but unable to provide emotional support during difficult times.

Male Friendships: Surface-Level Connections

Male friendships suffer significantly from Quiet BPD patterns because traditional masculine friendship norms discourage the emotional vulnerability required to move beyond surface-level connection.

You might notice patterns like:

- Having many acquaintances but few close friends
- Friendships that revolve around shared activities rather than emotional sharing
- Difficulty maintaining friendships during stressful periods
- Feeling like your male friends don't really know you
- Discomfort when other men share personal struggles or emotions
- Isolation during times when you most need support

The tragedy is that male friendship can provide crucial support for men's mental health, but BPD symptoms prevent you from accessing this support when you need it most.

Professional Relationships: Distant but Dependent

Work relationships often feel safer than personal relationships because they have clear boundaries and expectations. However, you may still struggle with the emotional regulation required for healthy professional relationships.

Common professional patterns include:

- Difficulty with criticism from supervisors or colleagues
- Intense reactions to workplace conflicts or office politics
- Either over-performing to prove your worth or under-performing due to emotional overwhelm
- Difficulty setting appropriate boundaries with colleagues
- Using work relationships to meet emotional needs that aren't being met personally

- Fear of professional rejection that affects job performance or career decisions

Breaking the Patterns

The relationship paradox of Quiet BPD isn't permanent. With awareness and appropriate tools, you can learn to tolerate the anxiety of intimacy without destroying the connections you crave. You can learn to communicate needs directly instead of testing them through behavior. You can develop the emotional regulation skills that make stable, satisfying relationships possible.

The key insights for changing relationship patterns include:

Understanding that your relationship fears are based on past experiences, not current reality. Your partner is not your father, mother, or previous partners who may have hurt or abandoned you.

Recognizing that testing behaviors create the very outcomes they're designed to prevent. Trust builds through positive experiences over time, not through surviving tests.

Learning that emotional vulnerability, while scary, is the foundation of authentic intimacy. You can't be loved for who you really are if no one knows who you really are.

Developing skills for emotional regulation that make intimacy less overwhelming. When you can manage your own emotional intensity, relationships become less threatening.

Building identity and self-worth that don't depend entirely on your relationships. When you have a stable sense of self, relationships become enhancing rather than essential for survival.

The desperate need for love doesn't have to be accompanied by terror of intimacy. **With the right understanding and tools, you can learn to move toward connection rather than alternately clinging and**

pushing away. The relationships you crave are possible when you develop the internal stability to sustain them.

Chapter 6: Professional Success as Survival Strategy

Your office is both your sanctuary and your prison.

Michael stares at the email marked "urgent" that came in at 9:47 PM. It's from his boss, asking for updates on the quarterly projections. Michael's already put in twelve hours today, but instead of irritation, he feels a familiar spike of anxiety. What if the delay means his boss is losing confidence in him? What if this is the beginning of being pushed out?

He opens his laptop and starts working, even though he knows the projections won't be needed until next week's meeting. By the time he finishes, it's 1:30 AM, and he's exhausted but somehow still wired with anxiety about tomorrow's performance.

This scene plays out nightly in Michael's life. Work has become both his identity and his prison. The office provides structure, validation, and a clear sense of worth through achievement. But it's also where he performs his most elaborate masking, where every interaction is carefully managed, and where his fear of failure creates impossible standards for himself.

For men with Quiet BPD, professional success often becomes the primary survival strategy - a way to prove worth, maintain identity, and avoid the chaos of internal emotional life.

The High-Functioning Facade

Perfectionism as Armor

Perfectionism in Quiet BPD isn't about having high standards - it's about believing that anything less than perfect performance will result in catastrophic rejection or failure. Every work project becomes a referendum on your worth as a person. Every mistake feels like evidence of fundamental inadequacy.

This perfectionism serves as psychological armor. If you can perform perfectly, no one can criticize you. If you can anticipate every possible problem, you can avoid the shame of being caught off-guard. If you can exceed every expectation, you can ensure that people value and need you.

But perfectionism as armor is exhausting and ultimately ineffective. The standards become impossible to maintain. The fear of imperfection creates paralysis around decision-making. The energy required to maintain perfectionist performance leaves nothing left for personal relationships or self-care.

Common perfectionist patterns include:

- Spending excessive time on projects that could be completed adequately with less effort
- Difficulty delegating because others might not meet your standards
- Procrastination on important tasks due to fear of imperfect execution
- Physical symptoms (headaches, insomnia, muscle tension) from constant pressure
- Inability to enjoy successes because you're already focused on the next potential failure
- Harsh self-criticism for normal human mistakes or limitations

Imposter Syndrome and the Fear of Exposure

Imposter syndrome affects many high achievers, but for men with Quiet BPD, it reflects a deeper fear that success is undeserved and that others will eventually discover you're fundamentally flawed or incompetent.

This fear of exposure creates constant vigilance. You monitor every interaction for signs that people are seeing through your professional competence. You over-prepare for meetings, second-guess decisions, and attribute successes to luck rather than skill.

The imposter syndrome in Quiet BPD often includes:

- Believing that past successes don't predict future performance
- Fear that current achievements are based on deception rather than genuine competence
- Anxiety that new challenges will expose your "real" limitations
- Difficulty accepting compliments or recognition
- Comparing your internal experience of uncertainty to others' apparent confidence
- Working harder than necessary to compensate for perceived inadequacies

This creates a vicious cycle: the harder you work to prove your competence, the more exhausted you become. The more exhausted you become, the more your performance actually suffers, which "confirms" your imposter fears.

Workaholism and Identity Fusion

For many men with Quiet BPD, work becomes fused with identity in ways that make it impossible to separate professional performance from personal worth. You don't just do your job - you are your job. Your title, responsibilities, and achievements become your entire sense of self.

This identity fusion creates several problems:

Vulnerability to professional setbacks: Normal work challenges feel like existential threats because they threaten not just your job, but your entire sense of who you are.

Difficulty with work-life balance: If work is your identity, then time away from work feels like time away from yourself. Vacations create anxiety rather than relaxation.

Relationship problems: Partners and family members compete with work for your attention, but work always wins because it feels more essential to your survival.

Physical and emotional burnout: Your body and mind weren't designed to maintain the constant activation required for workaholism.

Retirement anxiety: The prospect of eventually leaving work creates terror about losing your entire identity and purpose.

Burnout Cycles and Career Instability

Despite appearing highly successful, many men with Quiet BPD experience cycles of burnout that can lead to career instability. The intensity required to maintain perfectionist performance isn't sustainable long-term.

Burnout cycles often follow this pattern:

1. *Honeymoon phase*: New job or promotion feels perfect, provides renewed sense of worth and purpose
2. *Intensification phase*: Increased responsibilities and expectations trigger perfectionist responses
3. *Pressure phase*: Performance anxiety increases, work hours extend, personal life suffers
4. *Exhaustion phase*: Physical and emotional resources become depleted
5. *Crisis phase*: Performance actually decreases due to exhaustion, confirming fears about inadequacy
6. *Recovery phase*: Either job change (starting the cycle over) or intervention that addresses underlying patterns

These cycles can create a career pattern of frequent job changes, unexplained departures from positions that seemed perfect, or periods of high achievement followed by crashes.

Workplace Triggers and Responses

Criticism as Abandonment

For men with Quiet BPD, professional criticism triggers the same abandonment fears that relationship conflicts create. Feedback from supervisors, performance reviews, or even constructive suggestions from colleagues can feel like personal attacks or threats to your professional survival.

Common responses to workplace criticism include:

- Immediate anxiety or panic that feels disproportionate to the feedback
- Ruminating about critical comments for days or weeks
- Difficulty distinguishing between constructive feedback and personal attacks
- Defensive responses that escalate minor feedback into major conflicts
- Physical symptoms (insomnia, loss of appetite, headaches) following criticism
- Impulsive decisions like job searching or resigning in response to feedback

The intensity of these responses often surprises both you and your colleagues, who may have intended their comments as routine feedback rather than serious criticism.

Performance Reviews as Existential Threats

Annual performance reviews become particularly triggering events for men with Quiet BPD. What should be routine evaluations of job performance feel like trials where your entire worth as a person is being judged.

Performance review anxiety might include:

- Weeks of anticipatory anxiety before scheduled reviews
- Detailed preparation that goes far beyond what's necessary
- Difficulty sleeping in the days leading up to reviews
- Catastrophic thinking about possible negative feedback
- Physical symptoms during the review meeting
- Difficulty hearing positive feedback when any negative points are mentioned
- Post-review rumination about every comment or suggestion

Even positive reviews may not provide relief if you focus on areas for improvement rather than acknowledging successes.

Team Dynamics and Splitting

BPD includes a tendency toward "splitting" - seeing people, situations, or organizations as either all good or all bad. In workplace settings, this can create problems with team dynamics and collaborative relationships.

Workplace splitting might look like:

- Idealizing new supervisors or colleagues initially, then becoming disappointed when they prove human
- Seeing workplace conflicts in black-and-white terms rather than recognizing complexity
- Difficulty working with people you perceive as having criticized or rejected you
- Creating alliances and rivalries that may not reflect actual workplace dynamics

- Leaving positions when disillusionment sets in rather than working through normal workplace challenges
- Difficulty with reorganizations or changes that disrupt established relationships

Authority Conflicts and Control Issues

Relationships with authority figures at work can be particularly challenging for men with Quiet BPD. Supervisors may trigger both your need for approval and your fear of being controlled or rejected.

Common authority conflicts include:

- Alternating between people-pleasing and rebellious responses to supervision
- Difficulty with micromanagement or close oversight
- Taking normal managerial decisions as personal criticisms
- Fear of disappointing authority figures leading to over-commitment
- Resentment about feeling dependent on supervisors for validation
- Difficulty advocating for your needs or setting boundaries with demanding bosses

The Cost of Masking

Energy Depletion from Constant Performance

Maintaining your professional persona requires enormous amounts of energy. You're constantly monitoring your emotional expression, managing others' perceptions, and suppressing authentic reactions that might not be "appropriate" for the workplace.

This constant performance creates:

- Physical exhaustion that rest doesn't resolve

- Difficulty concentrating on actual work tasks due to energy spent on emotional management
- Reduced creativity and problem-solving ability when resources are depleted
- Increased irritability at home as your ability to regulate emotions becomes depleted
- Physical symptoms like headaches, muscle tension, and digestive issues
- Cognitive overload from simultaneously managing work tasks and emotional performance

After-Work Collapse and Isolation

Many men with Quiet BPD experience a significant "crash" when they get home from work. The mask that held you together all day suddenly feels impossible to maintain, but instead of relief, you experience emptiness, anxiety, or emotional overwhelm.

This crash often involves:

- Complete emotional withdrawal from family members
- Inability to engage in conversation about the day
- Need for isolation and recovery time that conflicts with family needs
- Using substances, food, or other behaviors to manage the transition
- Difficulty being emotionally available for children or partners
- Sleep disruption despite physical exhaustion

This pattern creates significant strain on personal relationships and prevents you from getting the support and connection you need to recover from workplace stress.

Substance Use for Decompression

Work-related stress and the exhaustion of constant masking often lead to increased substance use as a way to transition from "work mode" to "home mode." Alcohol, marijuana, or other substances provide temporary relief from the hypervigilance required for professional performance.

Workplace-related substance use might include:

- Daily alcohol use to "unwind" from work stress
- Increased consumption during high-pressure work periods
- Using substances to manage anxiety about work performance
- Drinking or using substances to fall asleep after stressful work days
- Weekend binge behaviors to recover from work week stress
- Hiding substance use from colleagues while maintaining perfect professional appearance

This creates additional problems as substances interfere with sleep quality, emotional regulation, and overall health, making work performance more difficult over time.

Physical Health Consequences

The chronic stress of maintaining a high-functioning facade while managing BPD symptoms takes a significant toll on physical health. The constant activation of stress response systems affects every system in your body.

Common physical health impacts include:

- Cardiovascular problems from chronic stress (high blood pressure, heart palpitations)
- Immune system suppression leading to frequent illnesses

- Digestive issues including stomach ulcers, acid reflux, or irritable bowel syndrome
- Sleep disorders that interfere with recovery and performance
- Chronic pain conditions, especially in the neck, shoulders, and back
- Skin problems that may be stress-related
- Weight gain or loss due to stress eating or loss of appetite

These physical symptoms often become additional sources of anxiety and can interfere with work performance, creating more stress and perpetuating the cycle.

Creating Sustainable Success

Identifying Values Beyond Achievement

Breaking free from the work-as-survival pattern requires identifying values and sources of meaning beyond professional achievement. This doesn't mean becoming less successful - it means creating a more balanced foundation for self-worth.

Questions for exploring broader values include:

- What did you care about before work became your primary identity?
- What would you want to be remembered for beyond your professional achievements?
- What activities or relationships give you energy rather than depleting it?
- How do you want to impact others' lives outside of work contexts?
- What would you do if you couldn't be defined by your career?

Developing a sense of self that includes but isn't limited to professional achievement creates resilience and reduces the existential threat of work challenges.

Setting Boundaries Without Guilt

Men with Quiet BPD often struggle with workplace boundaries because saying "no" feels like risking rejection or abandonment. Learning to set appropriate boundaries requires both practical skills and emotional regulation.

Effective workplace boundaries include:

- Reasonable limits on work hours that protect personal time and relationships
- Clear communication about your capacity and availability
- Saying no to additional responsibilities when your plate is already full
- Taking vacation time without checking email or doing work
- Asking for clarification about expectations rather than assuming unrealistic standards
- Advocating for resources you need to do your job effectively

Managing Emotional Reactions Professionally

Learning to manage BPD symptoms in professional settings requires developing specific skills for workplace emotional regulation. This isn't about suppressing all emotions - it's about responding appropriately to workplace triggers.

Strategies for workplace emotional regulation include:

- Taking breaks when you feel overwhelmed rather than pushing through
- Using brief mindfulness techniques to center yourself during stressful meetings

- Preparing responses to common triggers rather than reacting impulsively
- Seeking clarification when you interpret comments as personal attacks
- Using email for difficult communications when face-to-face feels too activating
- Having a trusted colleague who can provide reality checks about workplace situations

Asking for Accommodations Strategically

Under the Americans with Disabilities Act, mental health conditions including BPD may qualify for reasonable workplace accommodations. However, requesting accommodations requires careful consideration of your specific needs and workplace culture.

Potential accommodations might include:

- Flexible work schedules that account for therapy appointments
- Modified workspace arrangements that reduce overstimulation
- Written instructions for complex tasks when anxiety interferes with verbal processing
- Permission to take short breaks for emotional regulation
- Modified supervision styles that account for sensitivity to criticism
- Deadline extensions during particularly difficult periods

The key is requesting accommodations that genuinely improve your performance rather than simply making work easier.

Redefining Professional Success

Professional success doesn't have to come at the cost of your mental health, physical well-being, or personal relationships. **True success includes sustainable performance that allows for personal fulfillment and authentic relationships.**

This redefinition might include:

- Measuring success by impact and contribution rather than just hours worked
- Valuing collaboration and team success rather than individual achievement
- Finding meaning in work that aligns with your broader values and purpose
- Building professional relationships based on authenticity rather than performance
- Creating career paths that support rather than compete with personal well-being
- Using your professional skills to contribute to causes you care about

Your office can become a place where you contribute your genuine talents and skills rather than a stage where you perform an exhausting role. **The same intensity and dedication that created your professional success can be channeled into sustainable patterns that enhance rather than drain your life.**

The goal isn't to become less successful - it's to become successful in ways that support your overall well-being and allow for the authentic relationships and personal fulfillment that make success meaningful.

Chapter 7: Getting the Right Help - Beyond Misdiagnosis

"Stop treating the symptoms. Start healing the source."

The Diagnostic Maze: Why Your Pain Has Been Misunderstood

Marcus sat in his seventh therapist's office in five years, watching another well-meaning professional shuffle through his file. "Let's talk about your anger management issues," she began, completely missing the terror behind his rage. Like so many men with Quiet BPD, Marcus had been labeled everything except what he actually was: a man with an attachment disorder masquerading as antisocial behavior.

The statistics are staggering and infuriating. Men with BPD are misdiagnosed 73% of the time on their first clinical encounter. They're handed labels like "intermittent explosive disorder," "bipolar II," or "adjustment disorder with mixed disturbance of emotions and conduct" - clinical jargon that treats symptoms while ignoring the underlying emotional dysregulation that's destroying their lives from within.

Why Therapists Miss Male BPD:

The diagnostic bias isn't malicious - it's systemic. Most mental health professionals were trained on research conducted primarily with female subjects. The DSM-5 criteria for BPD were written with the "classic" presentation in mind: dramatic, externalized emotions, self-harm visible on the skin, relationship chaos that spills into public view.

But men? We've been conditioned since boyhood to internalize our chaos. Your self-harm isn't cutting - it's the third scotch every night, the 80-hour work weeks, the motorcycle rides at dangerous speeds on empty highways. Your "frantic efforts to avoid abandonment" don't look like begging someone to stay - they look like pushing them away before they can leave you first.

The Male BPD Presentation That Professionals Miss:

- **Anger as the only acceptable emotion:** While women with BPD might cry or plead, men learned early that anger is the only feeling that doesn't get you labeled as weak. Your rage isn't about control - it's about the terror of being left, abandoned, or revealed as fundamentally flawed.

- **Achievement as identity stabilization:** Instead of dramatic identity shifts, you've created a rigid professional persona that feels more real than who you are underneath. The successful executive, the respected father, the reliable friend - all masks covering an empty center.

- **Withdrawal instead of pursuit:** Classic BPD involves frantic efforts to avoid abandonment through pursuit. Male Quiet BPD avoids abandonment through preemptive withdrawal. You ghost relationships before they can ghost you.

- **Substance use as emotional regulation:** While cutting provides immediate physical relief from emotional pain, alcohol, drugs, or behavioral addictions serve the same function - they're your emotional anesthesia.

Breaking Through the Diagnostic Bias

Preparing for Your Assessment:

Before you walk into another professional's office, arm yourself with specific language. Don't say "I have anger issues." Say: "I experience intense rage that feels disproportionate to triggers, and underneath it is terror of being abandoned or rejected." Don't say "I work too much." Say: "I use achievement and work to regulate emotional states and maintain identity stability."

The Right Questions to Ask Potential Therapists:

1. "What experience do you have with personality disorders, specifically BPD in men?"
2. "How familiar are you with Quiet or High-Functioning BPD?"
3. "What's your approach to working with clients who present with anger but have underlying attachment trauma?"
4. "Do you use DBT skills, and how do you adapt them for male clients?"
5. "How do you work with clients who are high-achieving but emotionally dysregulated?"

Red Flags in Therapeutic Responses:

- "You don't seem like someone with BPD" (based on gender stereotypes)
- Immediate focus on anger management without exploring underlying fears
- Dismissing your relationship patterns as "just being male"
- Reluctance to consider personality disorders due to "stigma"
- Overemphasis on medication without addressing psychological factors

Treatment Approaches That Actually Work for Men

Dialectical Behavior Therapy (DBT) - Adapted for Male Sensibilities:

DBT was created by Marsha Linehan specifically for BPD, but traditional DBT groups can feel foreign to men who've spent decades avoiding emotional expression. Look for therapists who adapt DBT skills using masculine-friendly language:

- **Distress Tolerance** becomes "Crisis Management Training"
- **Emotion Regulation** becomes "Performance Optimization Under Pressure"
- **Interpersonal Effectiveness** becomes "Strategic Communication Skills"
- **Mindfulness** becomes "Situational Awareness Training"

The skills remain the same, but the framework helps you access them without feeling like you're violating your masculine identity.

Schema Therapy - Healing the Boy Inside the Man:

Schema Therapy directly addresses the childhood origins of your adult pain. It identifies the "modes" - the different parts of yourself that take control in different situations. For men with Quiet BPD, common modes include:

- **The Detached Protector:** The part that shuts down emotionally to avoid pain
- **The Angry Child:** The part that rages when feeling abandoned or criticized
- **The Punitive Parent:** The internal critic that's never satisfied
- **The Vulnerable Child:** The scared, lonely part you've learned to hide

Schema therapy helps you understand these parts without judgment and develop healthier ways of meeting their needs.

EMDR for Trauma Processing:

Many men with Quiet BPD have trauma histories that traditional talk therapy can't reach. Eye Movement Desensitization and Reprocessing (EMDR) allows you to process traumatic memories without having to verbally articulate experiences you may not even consciously remember.

Somatic Approaches - When Your Body Holds the Truth:

Years of emotional suppression create physical patterns in your body. Somatic therapies help you recognize how trauma and emotion manifest physically:

- That chronic back pain might be carrying the weight of unexpressed grief
- The jaw tension could be from years of "biting your tongue" emotionally
- The insomnia might be your nervous system's inability to feel safe enough to rest

Building Your Treatment Team

The Therapeutic Relationship:

Finding the right therapist is like dating - you need chemistry, trust, and mutual respect. Unlike dating, you're paying them to call you out on your patterns while creating a safe enough environment for you to be vulnerable. This is particularly challenging for men with Quiet BPD who've learned that vulnerability equals danger.

What to Look for in a Male BPD Therapist:

- Someone who can handle your anger without becoming defensive or trying to shut it down
- A professional who understands that your withdrawal isn't resistance - it's protection

- Someone who won't try to "fix" you quickly but can tolerate sitting with your pain
- A therapist who can challenge you without triggering your abandonment fears

Psychiatrist Collaboration:

Medication can be a valuable part of treatment, but it's not a cure. For men with Quiet BPD, certain medications can provide stability while you develop emotional regulation skills:

- **Mood stabilizers** can reduce the intensity of emotional swings
- **Antidepressants** may help with the chronic emptiness and depressive episodes
- **Anti-anxiety medications** (used carefully) can provide short-term relief during crisis periods

Important: No medication cures BPD. Pills can't teach you how to form secure attachments or regulate emotions effectively. They can, however, create enough stability for therapy to be effective.

Group Therapy Considerations:

Men often resist group therapy, but it's incredibly valuable for BPD recovery. Being witnessed by other men who understand your struggle breaks the isolation that keeps you sick. Look for:

- Men's therapy groups (if available)
- DBT skills groups with male-friendly facilitators
- Support groups specifically for personality disorders
- Online communities for men with BPD

Insurance and Practical Considerations

Navigating Insurance Coverage:

Personality disorder treatment is often poorly covered by insurance, but there are strategies:

- Get a primary diagnosis that insurance covers better (like depression or anxiety) while addressing BPD in treatment
- Look for therapists who offer sliding scale fees
- Consider intensive outpatient programs (IOPs) that may have better coverage
- Employee Assistance Programs (EAPs) through work often provide free initial sessions

The Investment Mindset:

Reframe therapy costs as an investment in your future earning potential, relationship satisfaction, and physical health. The cost of NOT treating BPD - in terms of career damage, relationship destruction, and physical health consequences - far exceeds the cost of treatment.

Crisis Resources You Need Now:

- National Suicide Prevention Lifeline: 988
- Crisis Text Line: Text HOME to 741741
- BPD-specific crisis line: Call your local NAMI chapter
- Your personalized crisis plan (we'll create this in Chapter 10)

Real Talk: What Recovery Actually Looks Like

Recovery from Quiet BPD isn't about becoming a different person - it's about becoming who you really are underneath all the protective strategies. You'll still be intense, passionate, and deeply feeling. The difference is you'll have skills to manage that intensity without it managing you.

What Changes:

- Your anger becomes information rather than a weapon
- Your work becomes meaningful rather than compulsive
- Your relationships become connections rather than performances
- Your solitude becomes peaceful rather than terrifying

What Stays the Same:

- Your drive and ambition (now aligned with your values)
- Your capacity for deep love and connection
- Your intuition and emotional intelligence
- Your ability to help others who are struggling

Remember: Seeking help isn't admitting weakness. It's the most courageous thing a man can do in a culture that teaches us suffering in silence is strength. Your willingness to get the right help is already evidence of the warrior spirit that will carry you through recovery.

Chapter 8: Emotional Intelligence for the Logical Mind

"Turn your analytical strength into emotional mastery."

Emotions as Data: The Engineer's Guide to Feelings

David stared at the spreadsheet on his laptop, tracking quarterly performance metrics with the precision he'd applied to everything in his professional life. Revenue up 23%, customer satisfaction scores improving, efficiency metrics all trending green. So why did he feel like he was drowning?

For the first time in his life, David realized he needed to apply the same analytical rigor to his internal experience that he brought to his external success. Emotions weren't mystical forces beyond understanding - they were data points, patterns to be recognized, systems to be optimized.

This chapter is specifically designed for the logical, analytical mind that rebels against "touchy-feely" approaches to emotional health. If you're a man who thinks in systems, processes, and metrics, this is your roadmap to emotional mastery using the cognitive strengths you already possess.

The Emotional Dashboard:

Think of emotions as your internal monitoring system - like the dashboard in your car that provides critical information about engine performance, fuel levels, and system status. You wouldn't ignore a check engine light, yet most men have been conditioned to ignore their emotional warning signals until complete system failure occurs.

Primary Emotional Metrics to Track:

1. **Intensity Level (0-10 scale):** How strong is this emotion right now?

2. **Duration:** How long has this feeling been present?

3. **Trigger Identification:** What specific event/thought preceded this emotional response?

4. **Physical Manifestation:** Where do you feel this in your body?

5. **Behavioral Urge:** What does this emotion make you want to do?

6. **Underlying Need:** What is this emotion trying to tell you?

Building Your Emotional Operating System

The STOP-LOOK-LISTEN-RESPOND Protocol:

When you notice emotional activation (anger, anxiety, sadness, emptiness), implement this four-step process:

STOP: Pause whatever you're doing. Create a brief circuit break between stimulus and response. This isn't about suppressing the emotion - it's about creating space for conscious choice rather than automatic reaction.

LOOK: Scan your internal state like running diagnostics on a system:

- What am I feeling right now? (Name it specifically)
- What's my intensity level? (Rate 1-10)
- Where do I feel this in my body? (Chest tightness, jaw clenching, stomach knots)

- What thoughts are running through my head? (Often catastrophic or all-or-nothing)

LISTEN: What is this emotion trying to communicate?

- Anger often signals boundary violations or threats to autonomy
- Anxiety usually indicates perceived danger or lack of control
- Sadness frequently points to loss or unmet needs
- Emptiness can signal disconnection from values or authentic self

RESPOND: Choose your action based on data rather than impulse:

- What would be most effective right now?
- What aligns with my long-term goals?
- How can I meet the underlying need this emotion is signaling?
- What would my best self do in this situation?

Emotional Regulation as System Optimization

The Three-Layer Approach:

Like any complex system, emotional regulation works on multiple levels simultaneously:

Layer 1: Hardware (Physical/Biological) Your body is the hardware running your emotional software. Optimize the basics:

- **Sleep Architecture:** 7-9 hours of quality sleep isn't optional - it's the foundation of emotional stability. Poor sleep amplifies emotional reactivity by 60%.
- **Nutritional Fuel:** Stable blood sugar prevents emotional volatility. Protein every 3-4 hours, complex carbohydrates, omega-3 fatty acids.

- **Movement Protocol:** 20-30 minutes of daily movement literally rewires your brain for better emotional regulation. Strength training, in particular, provides measurable confidence and stress resilience.

- **Recovery Systems:** Active recovery through breathwork, cold exposure, or meditation builds your capacity to handle emotional intensity.

Layer 2: Software (Cognitive/Mental) Your thoughts are the software running on your biological hardware:

- **Thought Auditing:** Track your automatic thoughts for patterns. Common male BPD thought distortions include: "I'm fundamentally flawed," "People will leave me if they really know me," "I have to be perfect to be acceptable."

- **Cognitive Restructuring:** Challenge catastrophic thinking with evidence-based analysis. Ask: "What evidence supports this thought? What evidence contradicts it? What would I tell a friend thinking this way?"

- **Reframing Protocols:** Transform emotional language into analytical language: "I'm losing my mind" becomes "I'm experiencing temporary emotional dysregulation that will pass."

Layer 3: Network (Social/Relational) Your relationships are the network your emotional system operates within:

- **Support System Architecture:** Map your current network. Who can you call at 2 AM? Who celebrates your successes? Who tells you hard truths? Identify gaps and build strategically.

- **Communication Protocols:** Develop scripts for difficult conversations. "I'm feeling overwhelmed and need to process this before responding" is more effective than exploding or withdrawing.

- **Boundary Management:** Clear boundaries aren't walls - they're property lines that define where you end and others begin.

Male-Friendly Regulation Techniques

Physical Strategies (For When Your Body Is the Problem):

Cold Exposure Protocol:

- Cold showers for 2-3 minutes daily build distress tolerance
- Ice baths for acute emotional crises (15-20 minutes provides 4-6 hours of emotional stability)
- The physiological reset helps when your nervous system is hijacked

Intensive Exercise:

- High-intensity interval training (HIIT) for anger management
- Heavy lifting for depression and emptiness
- Endurance cardio for anxiety and rumination
- Combat sports for controlled aggression release

Breathwork Systems:

- 4-7-8 breathing for acute anxiety (inhale 4, hold 7, exhale 8)
- Box breathing for general regulation (4-4-4-4 pattern)
- Wim Hof method for building stress resilience
- 2:1 exhale breathing for parasympathetic activation

Cognitive Strategies (For When Your Mind Is the Problem):

Evidence-Based Thinking: Apply the same critical thinking you use professionally to your emotional experiences:

- "What evidence do I have that this relationship is doomed?" (versus feeling like it's doomed)
- "What data supports the belief that I'm a failure?" (versus feeling like a failure)
- "What would a neutral observer see in this situation?" (versus your catastrophic interpretation)

Cost-Benefit Analysis: Before acting on emotional impulses, run a quick cost-benefit analysis:

- Short-term relief vs. long-term consequences
- Emotional satisfaction vs. relationship damage
- Immediate gratification vs. goal achievement

Scenario Planning: Use strategic thinking to manage emotional crises:

- Best case scenario: What's the most positive realistic outcome?
- Worst case scenario: What's the actual worst that could happen (not the catastrophic fantasy)?
- Most likely scenario: Based on evidence and experience, what will probably happen?
- Contingency plans: What will you do in each scenario?

From Rage to Response: Transforming Your Anger

Understanding Anger as Information:

For men with Quiet BPD, anger is often the only emotion we can access, but it's rarely the primary emotion. Anger is usually a secondary emotion - a protective response to more vulnerable feelings like fear, hurt, shame, or sadness.

The Anger Iceberg Analysis:

Surface emotion: Anger/Rage Underlying emotions might be:

- Fear (of abandonment, rejection, failure)
- Hurt (from criticism, dismissal, betrayal)
- Shame (feeling fundamentally flawed or unworthy)
- Sadness (from loss, disappointment, loneliness)

The 24-Hour Rule for Major Decisions:

When intense emotions are present, implement a mandatory 24-hour delay before making significant decisions or having important conversations. This isn't procrastination - it's quality control.

During the 24-hour period:

- Use physical regulation techniques to reduce emotional intensity
- Journal or voice-record your thoughts to externalize them
- Sleep on it (literally - sleep provides emotional perspective)
- Consult with trusted advisors if appropriate
- Revisit the situation when you can think clearly

Channeling Intensity Productively:

Your emotional intensity isn't a bug - it's a feature. The same passion that can destroy relationships can also fuel extraordinary achievement and deep connections when properly channeled:

- **Creative outlets:** Writing, music, art as emotional expression
- **Physical challenges:** Athletic goals, martial arts, adventure sports
- **Service work:** Helping others transforms personal pain into purpose

- **Professional intensity:** Channel emotional energy into meaningful work

Assertiveness Without Aggression

The Masculine Communication Paradox:

Most men with Quiet BPD swing between two extremes: aggressive communication (bulldozing others) or passive communication (disappearing entirely). Assertive communication is the middle path - expressing your needs clearly while respecting others' needs.

The DESC Script for Difficult Conversations:

Describe: State the situation objectively, without interpretation or judgment "When our dinner plans got cancelled last minute..."

Express: Share your emotional experience using "I" statements "I felt disappointed and unimportant..."

Specify: Request specific behavioral changes "In the future, I'd appreciate at least 2 hours notice if plans change..."

Consequences: Explain positive outcomes of change (not threats) "This would help me feel more valued and make our time together more enjoyable."

Managing Criticism Without Destruction:

Criticism feels like abandonment to the BPD brain, but it's often just information. Develop these responses:

- "Help me understand what you mean by that."
- "I can see you're frustrated. What specific change would help?"
- "I'm feeling defensive right now. Can we revisit this when I can listen better?"
- "What would success look like to you in this situation?"

Building Your Emotional Fitness Program

Daily Practices (The Emotional Workout):

Morning Check-in (5 minutes):

- Rate your emotional state (1-10)
- Identify any physical sensations
- Set an emotional intention for the day
- Choose one regulation tool to practice

Midday Reset (2 minutes):

- Brief body scan for tension
- Three deep breaths
- Adjust your approach based on current state
- Practice gratitude for one thing going well

Evening Review (10 minutes):

- What emotions did you experience today?
- What triggered intense feelings?
- How did you handle challenging situations?
- What would you do differently?
- What are you grateful for?

Weekly Emotional Analytics:

- Track patterns in your emotional intensity
- Identify your most common triggers
- Note which regulation techniques work best
- Celebrate progress and growth

- Adjust your approach based on data

Monthly System Optimization:
- Review your emotional fitness progress
- Update your crisis management plan
- Assess relationship quality and communication patterns
- Set new challenges for emotional growth
- Plan for upcoming stressful periods

Remember: Emotional intelligence isn't about becoming soft or losing your edge. It's about optimizing your human operating system for peak performance across all life domains. The same analytical skills that make you successful professionally can make you masterful emotionally - you just need to apply them systematically to your inner world.

Chapter 9: Building Connections That Heal

"Vulnerability isn't weakness - it's your superpower."

The Connection Paradox: Desperate for Love, Terrified of Intimacy

Jake's phone buzzed with another text from Sarah: "Are we still on for dinner tonight?" For most people, this would be a simple yes-or-no question. For Jake, it triggered a familiar spiral of contradictory impulses. Part of him craved the connection, the warmth of being with someone who cared about him. But another part - the part that had learned early that people always leave - wanted to cancel, to disappear before she could see too much, before she could discover he was fundamentally flawed and walk away like everyone else eventually did.

This is the core tragedy of Quiet BPD in men: You desperately need connection to heal, but connection feels like walking into a burning building. Every relationship becomes a paradox - the very thing you need most is the thing that terrifies you most.

Rewiring Attachment: From Fearful-Avoidant to Earned Security

Understanding Your Attachment Operating System:

Your attachment style isn't your destiny - it's your starting point. Think of it as the default settings on your relational software, programmed by early experiences but completely upgradeable with conscious effort.

Fearful-Avoidant Attachment in Men:

- You want close relationships but feel uncomfortable with too much closeness
- You tend to have a negative view of yourself and others
- You create distance when relationships become too intense
- You're hypervigilant for signs of rejection or abandonment
- You often feel like you're "too much" or "not enough" simultaneously

The Path to Earned Security:

"Earned security" means you can develop secure attachment patterns regardless of your childhood experiences. It requires understanding that your relational fears made perfect sense given your early experiences, but they don't serve you now.

Small Steps Toward Trust:

The 1% Rule: Instead of expecting yourself to become vulnerable overnight, commit to being 1% more open in each interaction. This might mean:

- Sharing one genuine feeling instead of defaulting to "fine"
- Asking for help with something small
- Expressing appreciation specifically instead of generally
- Admitting when you don't know something
- Showing up consistently for minor commitments

The Gradual Exposure Protocol: Like treating a phobia, you need to gradually expose yourself to increasing levels of emotional intimacy:

Level 1: Share factual information about yourself Level 2: Share preferences and opinions
Level 3: Share past experiences (non-traumatic) Level 4: Share

current struggles (low stakes) Level 5: Share fears and insecurities Level 6: Share childhood experiences and wounds Level 7: Share your deepest fears about the relationship itself

Managing Abandonment Fears:

The Evidence File: Keep a written record of evidence that contradicts your abandonment fears:

- Times people have stayed when things got difficult
- Relationships that ended for reasons unrelated to your "flaws"
- People who have consistently shown up for you
- Positive feedback you've received about your character
- Examples of your own loyalty and commitment to others

The Abandonment Fire Drill: When abandonment fears spike, use this protocol:

1. Pause and recognize this as your attachment system activating
2. Remind yourself: "This is my fear, not necessarily reality"
3. Look for actual evidence of abandonment versus perceived threats
4. Reach out for reality-testing with a trusted person
5. Take care of yourself as you would a frightened child
6. Stay present instead of fleeing or attacking

Tolerating Intimacy Incrementally:

The Intimacy Thermostat: Learn to recognize your optimal intimacy temperature. Too little connection leaves you empty and desperate. Too much triggers your flight response. The goal is finding your sweet spot and gradually expanding your comfort zone.

Signs You're at Your Intimacy Limit:

- Sudden urges to pick fights or create distance
- Feeling claustrophobic or trapped
- Wanting to run away or shut down
- Criticism of your partner that feels disproportionate
- Fantasizing about being single or with someone else

Healthy Responses to Intimacy Overwhelm:

- "I'm feeling overwhelmed and need some space to process this. Can we revisit this tomorrow?"
- "I care about you and I'm feeling scared right now. Help me understand what's happening."
- "This conversation is bringing up some old fears for me. I need a break but I want to come back to this."

Communication Renovation: From Defense to Connection

Speaking Feelings in "Man-Friendly" Language:

Many men struggle with emotional vocabulary because we were never taught the language. Start with these basic translations:

Instead of: "I'm fine" → "I'm processing something and need a few minutes" Instead of: "Whatever" → "I'm feeling dismissed and need to be heard" Instead of: "I don't care" → "I care so much it scares me" Instead of: "You're crazy" → "I don't understand your perspective, help me see it" Instead of: "Forget it" → "I'm feeling hurt and don't know how to express it"

The Emotional Weather Report:

Frame your internal experience like a weather report - describing current conditions without drama:

- "I'm experiencing some heavy emotional weather today"

- "There's a storm system moving through my head right now"
- "I'm in a fog and having trouble seeing clearly"
- "It's sunny with a chance of irritability this afternoon"

Active Listening Without Fixing:

This is perhaps the hardest skill for men to master. We're wired to solve problems, but sometimes people just need to be heard.

The WAIT Protocol:

- **W**hy am I talking? (Check your motivation)
- **A**m I trying to fix or just listen?
- **I**s this about them or about me?
- **T**ime to pause and really hear them

Listening Responses That Build Connection:

- "That sounds really difficult."
- "Help me understand more about that."
- "What was that like for you?"
- "I can see why you'd feel that way."
- "What do you need from me right now?"

Responses That Shut Down Connection:

- "At least..." (minimizing)
- "You should..." (fixing)
- "When I..." (redirecting to yourself)
- "That's nothing..." (comparing)
- "Just..." (oversimplifying)

Boundary Setting Without Building Walls

The Fence vs. Wall Distinction:

Healthy boundaries are like property fences - they clearly define where you end and others begin while still allowing for connection. Walls, on the other hand, shut everyone out completely.

Boundary Language That Works:

- "I'm not available for that, but here's what I can do..."
- "I need to think about that and get back to you."
- "That doesn't work for me. What other options do we have?"
- "I care about you and I can't rescue you from this situation."
- "I'm willing to discuss this when we can both stay calm."

Common Boundary Challenges for Men with Quiet BPD:

The Caretaker Trap: You try to manage everyone else's emotions to avoid abandonment, but end up resenting the very people you're trying to help.

The Isolation Solution: When boundaries feel too complicated, you withdraw entirely, missing out on connection and support.

The All-or-Nothing Approach: You either have no boundaries (letting people walk all over you) or walls so high nobody can reach you.

Healthy Boundary Scripts:

For work: "I check email until 7 PM on weekdays. After that, I'm focused on family time."

For family: "I love you and I can't be responsible for managing your anxiety about this decision."

For friends: "I value our friendship and I need you to respect when I say I need space."

For partners: "I want to be close to you and I need some autonomy to feel safe in our relationship."

Conflict Resolution Without Destruction

The BPD Conflict Cycle:

1. Trigger occurs (criticism, perceived rejection, unmet need)
2. Emotional dysregulation kicks in
3. Fight-or-flight response activates
4. You either explode (attack) or implode (withdraw)
5. Relationship damage occurs
6. Shame and regret set in
7. Desperate attempts to repair
8. Temporary resolution until next trigger

Breaking the Cycle:

The Circuit Breaker Approach: When you feel emotional intensity rising above a 7/10, implement an automatic pause:

"I can feel my emotions getting intense. I need 20 minutes to regulate myself so I can have this conversation in a way that's good for both of us."

The 24-Hour Rule for Relationship Conflicts: No major relationship decisions or conversations when emotions are above 7/10. Sleep, regulate, then engage.

The Repair Process:

Acknowledge: "I can see that my reaction hurt you." **Accept Responsibility:** "I'm responsible for how I responded, regardless of what triggered me." **Apologize:** "I'm sorry for [specific behavior], not for how you felt about it." **Amend:** "Here's what I'm going to do differently next time." **Ask:** "What do you need from me to help repair this?"

Relationship Rebuilding: From Performance to Partnership

Moving Beyond Transactional Relationships:

Many men with Quiet BPD create transactional relationships: "If I do X, then you'll stay." This turns love into a business deal instead of a genuine connection.

Signs of Transactional Relating:

- Keeping score of who did what
- Expecting specific returns on emotional investments
- Feeling resentful when your efforts aren't appreciated "enough"
- Believing love must be earned through performance
- Withdrawing affection when you don't get what you want

Building Genuine Partnerships:

Mutual Vulnerability: Both people share fears, dreams, and struggles without one person always being the "helper" or "helped."

Interdependence: You can rely on each other while maintaining individual identity and interests.

Unconditional Positive Regard: You accept each other's fundamental humanity while still having boundaries around behavior.

Growth Mindset: You see conflicts as opportunities to understand each other better, not as threats to the relationship.

Dating with BPD: The Disclosure Dilemma

When and How to Share Your Diagnosis:

There's no perfect timing, but here are general guidelines:

Too Early (Red Flags):

- First date emotional dumping
- Using your diagnosis to excuse bad behavior
- Leading with your mental health struggles

Too Late (Also Red Flags):

- After you're already living together
- After major emotional episodes without explanation
- When they discover it through other means

The Sweet Spot:

- When you're considering becoming exclusive
- After you've established some trust and connection
- When you can frame it as part of your growth story, not your identity

The Disclosure Script: "There's something I want you to know about me because I care about you and see potential for us. I have borderline personality disorder, which means I sometimes struggle with emotional regulation and relationships. I'm in therapy, I'm working on it actively, and I wanted you to understand this part of me rather than just wondering why I sometimes react intensely to things."

Creating Your Chosen Family

Beyond Blood Relations:

For many men with Quiet BPD, biological family relationships are complicated or toxic. Creating a "chosen family" of people who truly know and accept you becomes essential for healing.

Elements of Healthy Chosen Family:

- People who can handle your intensity without taking it personally
- Friends who celebrate your successes without jealousy
- Mentors who can guide you through challenges
- Peers who understand your struggles firsthand
- People you can call at 3 AM if needed

Building Your Support Network:

The Five-Person Rule: You need at least five people in your life who know about your BPD and support your recovery:

1. Your therapist or treatment provider
2. A best friend or close confidant
3. A romantic partner (current or potential)
4. A mentor or older male role model
5. A peer who understands mental health struggles

Network Maintenance:

- Regular check-ins, not just crisis calls
- Reciprocal support - you give as much as you receive
- Honest communication about your needs and limitations
- Appreciation expressed regularly
- Boundaries maintained to prevent burnout

The Vulnerability Paradox: Strength Through Openness

Redefining Masculine Vulnerability:

Vulnerability isn't about being weak or emotional. It's about having the courage to show up authentically when you can't control the outcome.

Masculine Models of Vulnerability:

- Warriors who admitted fear before battle
- Leaders who acknowledged their mistakes publicly
- Fathers who apologized to their children
- Athletes who discussed mental health struggles
- Businessmen who asked for help during crises

The Vulnerability Practice:

Start small and build your vulnerability muscles:

Week 1: Share one genuine preference instead of saying "I don't care" **Week 2:** Admit when you don't understand something **Week 3:** Ask for help with a small task **Week 4:** Express appreciation specifically and genuinely **Week 5:** Share a minor struggle you're working through **Week 6:** Admit a mistake without defensiveness **Week 7:** Express a need clearly and directly **Week 8:** Share something you're proud of without minimizing it

Remember: The goal isn't to become emotionally dependent or to overshare with everyone. The goal is to develop the capacity for genuine intimacy with safe people. Your relationships should enhance your life, not consume it. The men who heal from Quiet BPD don't become different people - they become more authentic versions of themselves. They keep their intensity, their passion, and their depth, but they learn to channel these gifts into connections that nourish rather than drain them.

Chapter 10: Your Daily Recovery Arsenal

"Consistency beats intensity in the recovery game."

The Recovery Operating System: Building Sustainable Habits

Marcus used to approach recovery like he approached everything else in his life - with intense bursts of effort followed by inevitable burnout. He'd meditate for two hours one day, then skip it for two weeks. He'd journal obsessively for a month, then abandon it when life got stressful. He'd commit to therapy twice a week, then cancel sessions when work demanded his attention.

The problem wasn't his commitment or motivation. The problem was treating recovery like a sprint when it's actually a marathon that never ends. Recovery from Quiet BPD isn't about dramatic breakthroughs or perfect days. It's about building a daily operating system that supports your emotional stability regardless of external circumstances.

This chapter provides you with a practical, male-friendly framework for daily recovery that works with your life, not against it. These aren't suggestions - they're requirements if you're serious about changing your life.

The Four Pillars of Daily Recovery

Think of your recovery as a building that needs four foundational pillars to remain stable:

1. **Physical Regulation** (Managing your nervous system)
2. **Emotional Processing** (Staying connected to your inner experience)
3. **Relational Connection** (Maintaining healthy relationships)
4. **Meaning and Purpose** (Living according to your values)

Neglect any one pillar and the entire structure becomes unstable. Maintain all four, and you create a foundation strong enough to weather any storm.

Pillar 1: Physical Regulation - Your Biological Foundation

The Morning Launch Sequence (20 minutes):

Your first 20 minutes awake determine your emotional trajectory for the entire day. This isn't optional self-care - it's essential system maintenance.

Minutes 1-5: Biological Optimization

- Hydrate immediately (16-20 oz of water)
- Expose yourself to natural light (even through a window)
- Take prescribed medications if applicable
- Three deep breaths to activate your parasympathetic nervous system

Minutes 6-10: Physical Activation

- 50 bodyweight exercises (pushups, squats, burpees - your choice)
- Cold shower for 2-3 minutes (builds distress tolerance)
- OR 5 minutes of yoga/stretching
- The goal is physiological activation, not exhaustion

Minutes 11-15: Mental Preparation

- Review your schedule and identify potential stress points
- Set one emotional intention for the day ("I will pause before reacting")
- Identify which emotional regulation tools you'll practice today

- Visualize handling one challenging situation calmly

Minutes 16-20: Connection

- Text one person something genuine (not just "good morning")
- Call a family member if appropriate
- Send an encouraging message to someone who needs it
- OR spend 5 minutes in grateful reflection

Workday Micro-Recoveries:

The 2-Minute Reset (every 2 hours):

- Stand up and do 10 deep breaths
- Quick body scan: Where am I holding tension?
- Drink water
- Ask yourself: "How am I doing emotionally right now?" (Rate 1-10)

The Bathroom Regulation Break: Use bathroom visits as regulation opportunities:

- 4-7-8 breathing (inhale 4, hold 7, exhale 8) three times
- Progressive muscle relaxation (tense and release major muscle groups)
- Positive self-talk: "I'm handling this well" or "This stress will pass"

Lunch Hour Recovery Protocol:

- Eat away from your desk/workspace
- Take a 10-minute walk outside if possible
- Listen to music that regulates your nervous system

- Call someone you care about (not work-related)
- Practice mindfulness while eating (taste, texture, temperature)

Evening Decompression Ritual (30 minutes):

Most men with Quiet BPD struggle with the transition from work mode to personal mode. You need a deliberate decompression protocol:

Minutes 1-10: Physical Transition

- Change clothes immediately when you get home
- Wash your hands and face (symbolic transition)
- Do 5 minutes of physical movement (walk, stretch, exercise)
- Put away work devices/materials

Minutes 11-20: Emotional Processing

- Rate your overall emotional state for the day (1-10)
- Identify the three most challenging moments
- Acknowledge what you handled well
- Release any anger/frustration through journaling or voice recording

Minutes 21-30: Connection and Preparation

- Connect meaningfully with family/roommates/partner
- Review tomorrow's schedule and prepare mentally
- Identify one thing you're grateful for today
- Set an intention for your evening activities

Pillar 2: Emotional Processing - Staying Connected to Your Inner World

The Daily Emotional Check-In:

Most men are taught to ignore emotions until they become unmanageable. Recovery requires daily emotional maintenance, like checking oil levels in your car.

Morning Emotional Assessment:

- Overall emotional state (1-10)
- Primary emotion present (anger, anxiety, sadness, emptiness, etc.)
- Physical sensations (where do you feel it in your body?)
- Underlying need (what is this emotion telling you?)

The RAIN Technique for Difficult Emotions:

When difficult emotions arise during the day, use the RAIN protocol:

Recognize: "I notice I'm feeling angry/scared/sad right now."
Allow: "It's okay to feel this way. This emotion is information."
Investigate: "Where do I feel this in my body? What triggered this?" **Non-identification:** "I am experiencing anger, but I am not my anger."

Weekly Emotional Intelligence Training:

Monday: Practice identifying emotions in real-time (set 5 phone alerts to check in) **Tuesday:** Focus on body awareness - notice physical sensations throughout the day **Wednesday:** Work on emotional vocabulary - use specific emotion words rather than "good," "bad," "fine" **Thursday:** Practice the opposite action skill - do the opposite of what your emotion urges you to do **Friday:** Focus on interpersonal effectiveness - practice expressing needs clearly **Saturday:** Work on distress tolerance - sit with difficult emotions without acting impulsively **Sunday:** Integration and planning - review the week and plan for upcoming challenges

Journaling for the Non-Journaler:

If traditional journaling feels too touchy-feely, try these masculine-friendly approaches:

The Daily Debrief:
- What went well today? (minimum 1 thing)
- What was challenging? (specific situation)
- What did I learn? (about myself or others)
- What will I do differently tomorrow? (one specific change)

Voice Recording:
- Record 5-10 minutes of thoughts while driving
- Talk through problems out loud
- Process emotions verbally rather than in writing
- Review recordings weekly for patterns

Bullet Point Processing:
- Use bullet points instead of paragraphs
- Focus on facts, feelings, and actions
- Rate intensity levels numerically
- Track patterns with symbols or colors

Pillar 3: Relational Connection - Maintaining Your Support Network

Daily Connection Requirements:

Isolation is toxic for BPD recovery. You need daily human connection, even when you don't feel like it.

The 1-3-7 Rule:

- 1 meaningful conversation daily (at least 10 minutes of genuine exchange)
- 3 people you check in with weekly (text, call, or in-person)
- 7 people in your broader support network you connect with monthly

Quality Connection vs. Social Performance:

Focus on authentic connection rather than social performance:

Authentic Connection:

- Sharing something genuine about your day/experience
- Asking questions because you actually care about the answer
- Being present and listening without planning your response
- Expressing appreciation specifically ("I appreciate how you...")
- Asking for help when you need it

Social Performance (Avoid):

- Going through motions without genuine engagement
- Pretending everything is fine when it's not
- Talking about yourself without showing interest in others
- Using conversations to manage your image
- Avoiding real topics in favor of surface-level chat

Crisis Connection Protocol:

When you're in emotional crisis (8+ on the intensity scale), you need a specific plan:

Immediate Response (First 30 minutes):

- Call your designated crisis person (identified in advance)

- Use physical regulation techniques while waiting for response
- Remove yourself from triggering environment if possible
- Remind yourself: "This is temporary, I will get through this"

Extended Support (First 24 hours):

- Stay connected with support people (don't isolate)
- Use grounding techniques and DBT skills
- Avoid major decisions or relationship conversations
- Focus on basic needs (food, sleep, safety)

Pillar 4: Meaning and Purpose - Living Your Values

Daily Values Alignment:

Recovery isn't just about managing symptoms - it's about building a life worth living aligned with your deepest values.

Values Identification Exercise: What matters most to you? Choose your top 5 from this list:

- Family relationships
- Professional excellence
- Personal growth
- Service to others
- Creative expression
- Physical health
- Financial security
- Adventure/new experiences
- Spiritual connection

- Learning and knowledge
- Independence/autonomy
- Community contribution

Daily Values Practice: Each morning, ask: "How will I honor my values today?" Each evening, ask: "How did I live my values today?"

The Legacy Question: Weekly, ask yourself: "If I continue living this way, what legacy will I leave? Is this aligned with who I want to be?"

Crisis Management: When Your System Breaks Down

The Emergency Protocol:

Even with daily practices, crises will occur. Having a plan prevents chaos from becoming catastrophe.

Crisis Identification (Rate 8-10 intensity):

- Thoughts of self-harm or suicide
- Uncontrollable rage or desire to hurt others
- Complete emotional numbness lasting more than 48 hours
- Inability to function in work/relationships
- Substance use to cope with emotions

Immediate Crisis Response:

1. **Safety First:** Remove means of self-harm, get to a safe environment
2. **Breathing:** 4-7-8 breathing for 5 minutes minimum
3. **Connection:** Call crisis person (not text)
4. **Professional Help:** Contact therapist, crisis line, or emergency services if needed

5. **Medication:** Take prescribed PRN medications if applicable

24-Hour Crisis Management:
- No major decisions for 24 hours
- Stay with supportive people if possible
- Focus only on basic needs (food, sleep, safety)
- Use intensive DBT skills every 2 hours
- Plan follow-up with treatment team

Crisis Recovery Protocol: After the acute crisis passes:
- Debrief with therapist about what triggered the crisis
- Identify early warning signs you missed
- Update your crisis plan based on what you learned
- Practice radical acceptance of your humanity
- Recommit to daily practices without shame

Technology Integration: Apps and Tools That Actually Help

Recommended Apps:
- **DBT Coach:** Daily skills reminders and practice
- **Insight Timer:** Meditation and sleep sounds
- **MyFitnessPal:** Food and mood tracking
- **Forest:** Focus and mindfulness
- **Headspace:** Guided meditations specifically for men

Digital Tracking Templates: Create simple spreadsheets to track:
- Daily emotional intensity (1-10)
- Sleep quality and duration

- Exercise completion
- Social connections made
- Medications taken
- Crisis episodes and triggers

Customizing Your System

Your Unique Recovery Profile:

Not every technique works for every person. Experiment and adapt:

High-Stress Profession: Focus more on micro-recoveries and stress inoculation **Relationship-Focused:** Emphasize communication skills and intimacy tolerance **Trauma History:** Include more somatic and grounding techniques **Substance Issues:** Add addiction-specific support and accountability **Physical Health Issues:** Adapt exercises and include medical team coordination

The 30-60-90 Day Build:

Days 1-30: Focus on morning and evening routines only **Days 31-60:** Add midday regulation and weekly emotional skills **Days 61-90:** Full integration of all four pillars

Quarterly System Reviews: Every three months, assess:

- What's working well?
- What needs adjustment?
- What new challenges have emerged?
- How can you upgrade your system?

Remember: This isn't about perfection. You'll miss days, skip practices, and have setbacks. The goal is consistency over time, not flawless execution. Recovery is a daily choice, not a destination. The men who succeed in recovering from Quiet BPD are the ones who show up for themselves daily, especially when they don't feel like it.

Your daily recovery arsenal isn't just about managing BPD symptoms - it's about building a life that's so fulfilling and stable that your old patterns naturally fall away. When you have effective tools for daily emotional regulation, meaningful connections with people who know and accept you, and a sense of purpose that gets you up in the morning, the chaos and emptiness of Quiet BPD become increasingly irrelevant to your daily experience.

This is how you go from surviving to thriving - one day, one practice, one choice at a time.

Chapter 11: For Partners, Families, and Allies

"Understanding without enabling, supporting without sacrificing."

For the Person Who Loves Someone with Quiet BPD

Sarah stared at her husband Michael as he silently ate breakfast, the familiar wall of distance growing between them like fog rolling in from the ocean. Yesterday they'd been planning a weekend getaway, laughing together as they looked at photos of mountain cabins. Today, after she'd made an innocent comment about wanting to invite another couple to join them, he'd withdrawn into that cold, unreachable space she'd come to dread.

"Did I do something wrong?" she'd asked, knowing the question would either be met with stony silence or an explosive "Nothing's wrong, I'm fine" that clearly meant everything was wrong. She loved this man deeply - his intelligence, his intensity, his capacity for loyalty and passion. But loving someone with Quiet BPD often felt like trying to embrace someone wearing armor while walking through an emotional minefield.

If you're reading this chapter, you're likely someone who cares deeply about a man with Quiet BPD. You might be a romantic partner, a parent, a child, a close friend, or a colleague who's noticed the patterns. This chapter is written specifically for you - to help you understand what's happening inside his mind, to give you tools for supporting his recovery without losing yourself in the process, and to help you navigate the unique challenges of loving someone whose emotional world operates by different rules than your own.

Understanding His Internal Reality

The Fear Behind the Anger:

When he explodes over something that seems minor to you, when he goes from zero to sixty in seconds, when his rage seems disproportionate to the trigger - understand that you're not seeing anger. You're seeing terror.

Inside his mind, your casual comment about changing dinner plans isn't just an inconvenience - it's evidence that you're losing interest, that he's not important enough for you to prioritize, that abandonment is imminent. His brain, wired by years of invalidation and attachment trauma, interprets neutral events as existential threats.

The Withdrawal Isn't About You:

When he suddenly becomes distant, when he stops sharing his day with you, when he seems to disappear emotionally while sitting right next to you - this isn't rejection of you. It's protection of himself.

His withdrawal is often a preemptive strike against the abandonment he's convinced is coming. In his mind, if he pulls away first, it will hurt less when you inevitably leave. If he stops needing you, stops depending on you, stops being vulnerable with you, then your departure won't destroy him.

This logic is flawed, but it's deeply embedded in his survival system. Understanding this can help you not take his withdrawal personally, even though it affects you deeply.

The Perfectionism Trap:

His relentless drive for achievement, his inability to accept "good enough," his tendency to work obsessively - these aren't just personality traits. They're desperate attempts to become worthy of love and acceptance.

In his mind, if he's successful enough, accomplished enough, useful enough, then maybe people will stay. Maybe he'll finally be enough. The tragic irony is that this perfectionism often pushes people away or prevents genuine intimacy, creating the very abandonment he's trying to prevent.

The All-or-Nothing Thinking:

To him, you're either completely for him or completely against him. A minor criticism becomes evidence that you don't love him. A small disappointment becomes proof that he can't count on you. A moment of distraction becomes abandonment.

This black-and-white thinking isn't intentional manipulation - it's how his brain processes information when his attachment system is activated. Gray areas feel too dangerous when you're convinced that people are either safe or threats, with no middle ground.

Supporting Recovery Without Losing Yourself

The Validation Paradox:

One of the most challenging aspects of supporting someone with BPD is learning to validate their emotional experience without agreeing with their distorted conclusions.

Validation Looks Like:

- "I can see you're really hurting right now."
- "It makes sense that you'd feel that way given your experience."
- "Your feelings are important to me, even when I don't understand them."
- "I want to help you through this."

Validation Does NOT Mean:

- Agreeing that you're actually abandoning him
- Accepting responsibility for his emotional state
- Changing your behavior to manage his emotions

- Pretending his perception of reality is accurate

Example: He says: "You don't love me anymore because you didn't text me back for two hours."

Unhelpful response: "That's ridiculous, of course I love you." (Invalidating his feeling)

Helpful response: "I can see you're feeling unloved and scared right now. Those feelings must be really painful. I was in meetings and couldn't respond, and I do love you very much."

Setting Loving Boundaries:

Boundaries aren't punishment - they're the structure that makes relationships sustainable. Without boundaries, supporting someone with BPD can consume your entire life.

Boundaries You Might Need:

- "I'm happy to talk about this when we can both stay calm."
- "I won't accept being yelled at or called names, regardless of how upset you are."
- "I need advance notice before changing plans, just like you do."
- "I can support you through this crisis, and I need you to also use your other coping tools."
- "I love you and I can't be responsible for managing your emotions."

The Boundary Script:

1. **Acknowledge their experience:** "I see that you're really struggling right now."
2. **State your boundary:** "I'm not willing to discuss this while voices are raised."

3. **Offer an alternative:** "I'm happy to revisit this conversation when we can both stay calm."
4. **Follow through:** If the boundary is violated, calmly disengage and try again later.

Encouraging Treatment Without Nagging:

Do:

- Express concern about specific behaviors: "I've noticed you seem to be struggling with sleep lately. How are you feeling about that?"
- Share how his wellbeing affects you: "When you're hurting, I hurt too. I want to support you in getting the help that might make you feel better."
- Offer practical support: "Would it help if I drove you to therapy appointments?" or "I can help you research therapists if you want."
- Acknowledge his efforts: "I've noticed you've been working really hard on using those breathing techniques. It shows."

Don't:

- Diagnose or label: "You're being borderline right now."
- Threaten ultimatums unless you mean them: "Get therapy or I'm leaving."
- Make his treatment your responsibility: Don't call his therapist, schedule his appointments, or manage his medication unless specifically asked.
- Compare him to others: "My friend's husband went to therapy and he's so much better now."

Managing Your Own Emotional Response

The Emotional Contagion Effect:

Living with or loving someone with intense emotions can cause you to absorb their emotional state. You might find yourself walking on eggshells, constantly monitoring his mood, or feeling anxious when he's anxious.

Protecting Your Emotional Space:

- Practice grounding techniques when his emotions feel overwhelming
- Remind yourself: "His feelings are his to manage, mine are mine to manage"
- Take regular breaks from emotional intensity
- Maintain your own routine and interests regardless of his emotional state

Avoiding the Caretaker Trap:

It's natural to want to help someone you love, but taking responsibility for their emotions creates an unhealthy dynamic that actually prevents their recovery.

Signs You've Become a Caretaker:

- You feel responsible for his mood
- You modify your behavior to prevent his emotional reactions
- You feel guilty for having your own needs or problems
- You make excuses for his behavior to others
- You feel exhausted from managing his emotional crises

Healthy Support vs. Caretaking:

Healthy Support:

- Offering comfort without trying to fix his emotions
- Maintaining your own life and interests

- Encouraging his independence and coping skills
- Setting boundaries around what you will and won't do

Caretaking:

- Trying to prevent all situations that might upset him
- Sacrificing your own needs to manage his emotions
- Making decisions for him to avoid conflict
- Taking blame for his emotional reactions

Communication Strategies That Work

De-escalation Techniques:

When emotions are running high, your goal is to reduce intensity, not to be right or to solve the problem immediately.

The LEAP Method:

- **L**isten without defending or explaining
- **E**mpathize with his emotional experience
- **A**sk questions to understand better
- **P**ause before responding

Phrases That De-escalate:

- "Help me understand what you're feeling right now."
- "That sounds really difficult."
- "What would be most helpful for you right now?"
- "I can see this is important to you."
- "Let's take a break and come back to this when we're both calmer."

Phrases That Escalate:

- "You're overreacting."
- "That's not what I meant."
- "You always..." or "You never..."
- "Calm down."
- "That's not what happened."

Timing Conversations:

Good Times to Talk:

- When emotions are at moderate levels (5/10 or below)
- After he's used regulation techniques
- When you're both well-rested and fed
- In private, comfortable settings
- When there's adequate time for the conversation

Bad Times to Talk:

- During or immediately after emotional crises
- When either of you is tired, hungry, or stressed
- In public or around others
- When rushing to get somewhere
- Late at night when emotions tend to be more intense

Family Dynamics and Children

If You Have Children Together:

Children in families affected by BPD need special consideration. They're often hypervigilant to emotional changes and may blame themselves for conflicts.

Age-Appropriate Explanations:

Ages 3-7: "Daddy sometimes has big feelings that are hard for him to handle. It's not your fault, and you're safe."

Ages 8-12: "Dad has something called an emotional disorder, which means his feelings get very intense sometimes. He's working with a doctor to get better. This isn't about you, and you don't need to fix it."

Ages 13+: "Your father has borderline personality disorder, which affects how he processes emotions and relationships. He's in treatment, and we're all learning how to handle this as a family."

Protecting Children from Emotional Chaos:

- Maintain consistent routines regardless of his emotional state
- Don't ask children to manage or fix his emotions
- Provide them with their own counseling if needed
- Ensure they have other stable adult relationships
- Be honest about what's happening without oversharing details

Family Meeting Guidelines:

Regular family meetings can help everyone understand expectations and feel heard:

- Set ground rules about respectful communication
- Allow everyone to express concerns safely
- Problem-solve together rather than making unilateral decisions
- Focus on specific behaviors rather than personality traits
- End meetings on positive notes when possible

Self-Care for Supporters

You Need Your Own Support System:

Supporting someone with BPD is emotionally demanding. You need people in your life who support you, not just advice about how to better support him.

Building Your Support Network:

- Individual therapy for yourself
- Support groups for families of people with mental illness
- Trusted friends who understand your situation
- Family members who can provide perspective
- Online communities for BPD family members

Warning Signs of Caregiver Burnout:

- Chronic exhaustion that sleep doesn't fix
- Resentment toward him or the situation
- Loss of interest in your own hobbies and relationships
- Feeling hopeless about the future
- Physical symptoms (headaches, stomach problems, sleep issues)
- Increased use of alcohol or other substances to cope

Essential Self-Care Practices:

- Regular exercise and sleep
- Hobbies and interests outside the relationship
- Social connections independent of him
- Professional support (therapy, coaching, medical care)
- Spiritual or meditative practices if meaningful to you

When Professional Help is Needed

Crisis Situations That Require Immediate Action:

- Threats of suicide or self-harm
- Threats to harm others
- Substance abuse that creates safety concerns
- Inability to function in work or daily life for extended periods
- Physical violence or destruction of property

Resources for Immediate Crisis:

- National Suicide Prevention Lifeline: 988
- Crisis Text Line: Text HOME to 741741
- Local emergency services: 911
- Your local hospital emergency room
- Mobile crisis response teams (if available in your area)

Encouraging Professional Help:

- Focus on specific, observable behaviors rather than labels
- Express your concerns from a place of love, not frustration
- Offer to help research therapists or attend first appointments
- Share how his wellbeing affects the family
- Be patient - readiness for treatment often takes time

Long-term Relationship Considerations

Recovery is Possible, But It Takes Time:

BPD recovery is typically measured in years, not months. There will be setbacks, challenging periods, and times when progress feels stalled. This doesn't mean he's not trying or that treatment isn't working.

Realistic Expectations:

- Emotional intensity may remain, but emotional regulation improves
- Relationship patterns change gradually, not overnight
- Trust rebuilds slowly after years of damaged attachment
- His core personality strengths remain - intensity, passion, loyalty
- Recovery enhances who he is rather than fundamentally changing him

Signs of Recovery Progress:

- Taking responsibility for his actions without excessive shame
- Using coping skills during emotional distress
- Maintaining employment or daily functioning more consistently
- Communicating needs and feelings more directly
- Showing empathy for how his behavior affects others
- Building and maintaining friendships outside the relationship

When to Consider Ending the Relationship:

This is never an easy decision, but sometimes it becomes necessary:

- When there's ongoing physical violence or credible threats
- When substance abuse takes priority over treatment
- When he consistently refuses to engage in treatment

- When your physical or mental health is seriously compromised
- When children are being significantly harmed by the emotional environment

Remember: You can love someone and still need to protect yourself. Staying in a relationship that's destroying your wellbeing doesn't help either of you recover.

Hope for the Future

What Recovery Looks Like for Families:

Families where someone has successfully managed BPD often describe their relationships as deeper and more authentic than before treatment. The intensity that once felt destructive becomes passion channeled into positive pursuits. The sensitivity that once created chaos becomes empathy and emotional intelligence.

Your Role in His Recovery:

You cannot cure his BPD, but you can:

- Model healthy emotional regulation
- Maintain your own stability and wellbeing
- Provide consistent, boundaried support
- Celebrate progress without taking credit for it
- Continue growing and healing yourself

The Parallel Process:

Often, when someone with BPD begins recovery, their family members also experience growth. You may discover your own patterns, heal your own childhood wounds, and develop emotional skills you never knew you needed.

Building a New Relationship:

Recovery isn't about returning to how things used to be - it's about building something new and healthier. This requires patience, courage, and commitment from everyone involved.

The relationship you build with someone recovering from BPD can be extraordinary in its depth, authenticity, and resilience. You'll both know you've weathered real storms together and chosen to keep building something beautiful despite the challenges.

Your love and support matter tremendously in his recovery, but remember: you're not responsible for fixing him, and you can't love him into wellness. What you can do is love him while he learns to love himself, support him while he develops his own strength, and maintain your own health while he works toward his own.

That's not just enough - that's everything.

Chapter 12: From Surviving to Thriving - Your Future Self

"Recovery isn't about becoming someone else - it's about becoming who you really are."

The Transformation: Who You're Becoming

David sat in his car outside his son's school, waiting for pickup and reflecting on a conversation he'd had with his therapist that morning. "Two years ago," she'd said, "you would have interpreted your boss's criticism as evidence that you were fundamentally flawed and probably about to be fired. Yesterday, you heard it as information about how to improve a presentation. What changed?"

What changed? Everything and nothing. He was still David - still intense, still passionate, still deeply feeling. But the intensity that once felt like a curse had become his greatest asset. The emotional depth that once threatened to drown him now allowed him to connect with people in ways that amazed him. The sensitivity that once made him feel broken now made him an incredible father, friend, and leader.

Recovery from Quiet BPD doesn't mean becoming emotionally flat or losing your edge. It means learning to channel your intensity into creation rather than destruction, connection rather than isolation, growth rather than survival.

Post-Traumatic Growth: Finding Meaning in the Struggle

The Phoenix Process:

Recovery from BPD is fundamentally a process of post-traumatic growth. You're not just healing from your wounds - you're discovering strengths and capabilities you never knew you possessed. The same sensitivity that made you vulnerable to emotional pain also makes you extraordinarily attuned to others' needs. The intensity that felt overwhelming now fuels passion projects and deep commitments.

Strengths Forged in Suffering:

Emotional Intelligence Beyond Measure: Your years of emotional chaos weren't wasted - they were graduate-level training in understanding human psychology. You can read emotional subtext that others miss entirely. You understand motivation, fear, and desire in ways that make you an extraordinary leader, friend, and partner.

Resilience That Can't Be Taught: You've survived emotional storms that would break many people. This isn't theoretical resilience - it's battle-tested strength. When life hits you with challenges, you have a deep knowing that you can survive and even thrive through difficulty.

Authenticity as a Superpower: Years of wearing masks taught you the cost of inauthenticity. In recovery, you develop the courage to show up genuinely in a world full of performative relationships. This authenticity attracts people who value real connection over surface-level interactions.

Capacity for Deep Love: Your intensity in relationships, once a source of chaos, becomes a capacity for love that's rare and precious. You don't love halfway - you love completely, passionately, loyally. In recovery, this becomes one of your greatest gifts to the world.

Intuitive Understanding of Pain: Your intimate familiarity with suffering makes you extraordinarily capable of helping others through their darkest moments. You don't offer platitudes or empty encouragement - you offer real understanding and hope based on lived experience.

Identity Beyond the Disorder

Who Are You When You're Not Defined by Your Symptoms?

One of the most profound aspects of BPD recovery is discovering who you are underneath the disorder. For years, your identity may have been built around your symptoms, your struggles, your chaos. Recovery requires rebuilding identity from the ground up.

Values-Based Identity:

Instead of "I am someone with BPD," you become "I am someone who values..."

- Deep, authentic relationships
- Excellence and craftsmanship in my work
- Growth and continuous learning
- Service to others who are struggling
- Creativity and self-expression
- Adventure and new experiences
- Family and legacy
- Justice and fairness
- Beauty and artistry
- Spiritual connection and meaning

Role-Based Identity:

You're not just a patient or someone in recovery. You're:

- A father raising children who feel truly seen and understood
- A professional whose intensity drives innovation and excellence
- A friend who can be counted on in any crisis
- A partner capable of intimacy that most people only dream about

- A mentor helping other men navigate their own emotional journeys
- A leader who creates psychologically safe environments for others
- A creative whose work reflects deep emotional truth

Characteristic-Based Identity:

Your core characteristics aren't symptoms to be managed - they're strengths to be channeled:

- Intense → Passionate and committed
- Sensitive → Empathetic and intuitive
- Emotional → Authentic and expressive
- All-or-nothing → Dedicated and thorough
- Reactive → Responsive and engaged
- Deep → Thoughtful and philosophical

Sustainable Recovery: Making It Last

Understanding Recovery as a Practice, Not a Destination:

Recovery isn't something you achieve once and then maintain passively. It's a daily practice, like physical fitness. Some days you'll feel strong and capable. Other days you'll struggle. Both are normal parts of the long-term process.

The Recovery Lifestyle:

Physical Foundation:

- Regular exercise that you actually enjoy (not exercise as punishment)
- Nutrition that supports stable mood and energy
- Sleep hygiene that prioritizes quality rest

- Medical care that addresses your whole person
- Substance use that enhances rather than numbs your life

Emotional Foundation:
- Daily emotional check-ins and regulation practices
- Weekly therapy or deep personal work
- Monthly goal-setting and values alignment
- Quarterly life reviews and course corrections
- Annual intensive retreats or workshops for deeper growth

Relational Foundation:
- Daily meaningful connections with people who matter
- Weekly quality time with your closest relationships
- Monthly reach-outs to broader network of friends and family
- Quarterly relationship check-ins to address any issues
- Annual recommitment to the people and communities you value most

Spiritual/Meaning Foundation:
- Daily practices that connect you to something larger than yourself
- Weekly engagement with activities that reflect your deepest values
- Monthly service or contribution to causes you care about
- Quarterly reflection on your life's direction and purpose
- Annual visioning and goal-setting for meaningful growth

Relapse Prevention: When Old Patterns Resurface

Understanding Relapse vs. Lapse:

A **lapse** is a temporary return to old patterns - maybe you withdraw for a few days during stress, or you have an emotional outburst during a conflict. This is normal and expected in recovery.

A **relapse** is a sustained return to pre-recovery functioning - stopping therapy, isolating completely, returning to destructive coping mechanisms, losing the ability to maintain work or relationships.

Early Warning Signs:

Red Flag Indicators:

- Sleep patterns disrupting (too much or too little)
- Increased irritability or emotional numbness
- Withdrawing from supportive relationships
- Skipping therapy or abandoning helpful practices
- Using work, substances, or other behaviors to avoid emotions
- Catastrophic thinking becoming dominant again
- Feeling like recovery "isn't worth it" or "isn't working"

The Relapse Prevention Protocol:

When You Notice Warning Signs:

1. **Acknowledge without judgment:** "I notice I'm struggling right now, and that's okay."
2. **Reach out immediately:** Call therapist, trusted friend, or support person
3. **Return to basics:** Focus only on essential daily practices

4. **Remove unnecessary stressors:** Simplify your life temporarily
5. **Increase support:** More therapy, more connection, more structure
6. **Practice radical acceptance:** This is part of the process, not evidence of failure

The Spiral Prevention Plan:

Create a written plan for when you notice yourself slipping:

- Three people you commit to calling when struggling
- Five specific skills you'll use when emotions get intense
- Your therapist's crisis contact information
- A list of activities that reliably help you feel grounded
- Reminders of why recovery matters to you
- Evidence of past recovery successes to review

Giving Back: From Wounded Healer to Healer

The Service Imperative:

One of the most powerful aspects of BPD recovery is the ability to help others who are suffering in similar ways. Your lived experience becomes a gift you can offer to others walking the same difficult path.

Ways to Give Back:

Peer Support:

- Facilitate or participate in BPD support groups
- Mentor other men early in their recovery journey
- Share your story in appropriate settings to reduce stigma

- Volunteer with mental health organizations
- Write about your experience to help others feel less alone

Professional Development:
- Train mental health professionals about male BPD presentation
- Consult with organizations about male mental health initiatives
- Speak at conferences or workshops about recovery
- Develop resources specifically for men with BPD
- Advocate for better mental health services and policies

Family and Community:
- Model emotional health for your children and partner
- Create psychologically safe environments in your workplace
- Support other families dealing with mental health challenges
- Normalize conversations about men's emotional wellbeing
- Challenge toxic masculinity in your social circles

Creative Expression:
- Write books, blogs, or articles about your experience
- Create art, music, or other expressions that reflect your journey
- Use your professional skills to benefit mental health causes
- Develop apps, resources, or tools that would have helped you
- Tell your story through whatever medium feels authentic

Your New Life: What Thriving Actually Looks Like

Authentic Success Redefined:

Success is no longer about perfection, external validation, or avoiding all emotional pain. Success becomes about:

Aligned Achievement: Your professional success flows from your values rather than fear. You excel because you care deeply about your work, not because you're terrified of failure. You can receive criticism without spiraling, celebrate victories without imposter syndrome, and find meaning in your contribution beyond just personal advancement.

Emotional Mastery: You still feel deeply, but emotions become information rather than emergencies. You can sit with sadness without being consumed by it. You can feel anger without destroying relationships. You can experience anxiety without avoiding all risk. Your emotions enhance your life rather than running it.

Relationship Depth: Your relationships are characterized by genuine intimacy rather than performance or crisis. People feel safe being authentic with you because you've learned to be authentic with yourself. Your capacity for love is no longer limited by your terror of abandonment.

Physical Vitality: Your body is no longer a battlefield where emotions play out through illness, tension, and exhaustion. You sleep well, eat nourishing foods, and move your body in ways that feel good. Physical wellness supports emotional wellness in an upward spiral.

Creative Expression: Whether through work, hobbies, or relationships, you express your authentic self regularly. The intensity that once felt destructive now fuels creativity, innovation, and passionate engagement with life.

Spiritual Connection: You have a sense of purpose that extends beyond your own immediate needs. This might be religious faith, connection to nature, service to others, or simply a deep appreciation for the mystery and beauty of existence.

Legacy: What You Leave Behind

The Generational Impact:

Your recovery doesn't just change your life - it changes the trajectory of your family line. Children who grow up with an emotionally healthy father learn that:

- Feelings are manageable and informative
- Relationships can be safe and nourishing
- Men can be both strong and vulnerable
- Intensity is a gift when properly channeled
- Recovery and growth are always possible

Breaking the Cycle:

Many men with BPD come from families where emotional dysregulation, trauma, and dysfunctional relationships were passed down through generations. Your recovery breaks that cycle. Your children will have struggles, but they won't have your struggles. They'll have an emotionally intelligent father who can teach them skills you had to learn as an adult.

Professional Legacy:

Your emotional intelligence, hard-won through years of struggle and recovery, makes you an exceptional leader, colleague, and innovator. You create workplaces where people feel psychologically safe. You mentor younger professionals not just in technical skills but in emotional resilience. Your career becomes about contribution, not just achievement.

Community Impact:

Your willingness to be open about mental health, to model emotional intelligence, and to support others who are struggling creates ripple effects throughout your community. Other men feel permission to seek help. Families learn that recovery is possible. Stigma decreases as people see successful, accomplished men who also happen to have mental health challenges.

Letter to Your Future Self

Take a moment to write a letter to the man you're becoming. What do you want to tell him? What do you want to thank him for? What do you want him to remember about this journey?

Dear Future Me,

If you're reading this, it means you made it through the hardest part. You survived the chaos, learned to regulate the storms, and discovered who you really are underneath all the protective strategies. I'm proud of you for not giving up when it felt impossible.

Remember that your sensitivity is not a weakness - it's your superpower. Your intensity is not a flaw - it's your fuel. Your depth is not a burden - it's your gift to the world.

The relationships you have now - the deep, authentic connections you've built - they exist because you had the courage to be vulnerable, to do the work, to show up imperfectly but consistently. The peace you feel now exists because you learned to make friends with your own mind.

Don't forget the men who are still struggling in the darkness you once knew. Your story matters. Your recovery matters. Your willingness to reach back and help others climb out of the pit matters more than you know.

Keep growing. Keep feeling. Keep connecting. Keep creating. The world needs what you have to offer.

With deep respect and gratitude, The man you used to be

The Continuing Journey

Recovery is Not a Destination:

There is no finish line where you suddenly become "cured" of BPD. Recovery is an ongoing process of growth, discovery, and choice. You'll have challenging days, difficult seasons, and unexpected setbacks. You'll also have moments of profound joy, deep connection, and authentic success that you never could have imagined during your darkest periods.

The Daily Choice:

Every morning, you wake up with a choice: Will you show up as the man you're becoming, or will you revert to old patterns? Recovery is the daily choice to:

- Feel your emotions without being controlled by them
- Connect with others despite the risk of rejection
- Pursue your values despite the possibility of failure
- Trust that you are worthy of love and belonging
- Believe that your story can inspire and help others

Your Story Continues:

This book ends, but your story continues. You are writing new chapters every day - chapters of healing, growth, love, and contribution. Your journey from the silent struggle of Quiet BPD to the authentic strength of recovery is not just personal transformation - it's a gift to everyone whose life you touch.

The man reading these words right now - whether you're just beginning to recognize yourself in these pages or you're years into your recovery journey - you have everything you need to create a life that's not just survivable, but genuinely thriving.

Your intensity is needed in this world. Your sensitivity is a gift waiting to be shared. Your capacity for deep feeling and authentic connection is exactly what our disconnected world desperately needs.

You are not broken. You never were. You were wounded, and you survived, and now you're healing. And in your healing, you give permission for other men to heal too.

The silent struggle is ending. The authentic life is beginning.

Welcome home to yourself.

EPILOGUE: A Message from the Author

If you've made it to this final page, you've taken a journey that requires tremendous courage. Whether you picked up this book because you recognized yourself in the description of Quiet BPD, or because someone you love is struggling with these patterns, you've confronted truths that our culture often makes men bury and ignore.

The statistics I shared in the opening chapters are not just numbers - they represent real men who suffered in silence, who never got the help they needed, who never learned that their struggles had a name and a path toward healing. By reading this book, by being willing to consider that there might be another way to live, you've already separated yourself from those statistics.

Recovery from Quiet BPD is not about becoming a different person. It's about becoming more fully yourself - accessing the parts of your personality that have been buried under years of protective strategies, discovering the strength that comes from emotional honesty, and learning to channel your intensity into connection and creation rather than isolation and destruction.

The journey is not easy. There will be setbacks, difficult conversations, moments when you question whether the work is worth it. In those moments, remember: You are not just healing yourself. You are breaking generational patterns, modeling emotional courage for other men, and contributing to a world where sensitivity and strength can coexist.

Your story matters. Your recovery matters. Your willingness to feel deeply and love authentically in a world that often demands emotional numbness from men is an act of rebellion and healing.

You are not alone in this struggle, and you are capable of the life you're working toward.

The silent struggle ends with you.

For resources, support communities, and additional tools for recovery, visit [website]. If you're in crisis, please reach out immediately to the National Suicide Prevention Lifeline at 988 or your local emergency services.

This book is dedicated to every man who has ever felt "too much" and "not enough" at the same time. Your intensity is not a flaw to be fixed - it's a strength to be channeled.

References

1. Addis, M. E., & Mahalik, J. R. (2003). Men, masculinity, and the contexts of help seeking. *American Psychologist, 58(1),* 5-14.

2. Ainsworth, M. D. S., Blehar, M. C., Waters, E., & Wall, S. (1978). *Patterns of attachment: A psychological study of the strange situation.* Lawrence Erlbaum Associates.b

3. American Psychiatric Association. (2022). *Diagnostic and statistical manual of mental disorders* (5th ed., text rev.). American Psychiatric Publishing.p

4. Bartholomew, K., & Horowitz, L. M. (1991). Attachment styles among young adults: A test of a four-category model. *Journal of Personality and Social Psychology, 61(2),* 226-244.i

5. Blazina, C., & Watkins Jr, C. E. (1996). Masculine gender role conflict: Effects on college men's psychological well-being, chemical substance usage, and attitudes toward help-seeking. *Journal of Counseling Psychology, 43(4),* 461-465.

6. Bowlby, J. (1988). *A secure base: Parent-child attachment and healthy human development.* Basic Books

7. Chapman, A. L., & Gratz, K. L. (2007). *The borderline personality disorder survival guide: Everything you need to know about living with BPD.* New Harbinger Publications.

8. Cochran, S. V., & Rabinowitz, F. E. (2000). *Men and depression: Clinical and empirical perspectives.* Academic Press.

9. Courtenay, W. H. (2000). Constructions of masculinity and their influence on men's well-being: A theory of gender and health. *Social Science & Medicine, 50*(10), 1385-1401.

10. Dutton, D. G., Saunders, K., Starzomski, A., & Bartholomew, K. (1994). Intimacy-anger and insecure attachment as precursors to abuse in intimate relationships. *Journal of Applied Social Psychology, 24*(15), 1367-1386.

11. Englar-Carlson, M., & Stevens, M. A. (2006). *In the room with men: A casebook of therapeutic change*. American Psychological Association.

12. Fonagy, P., Gergely, G., Jurist, E., & Target, M. (2018). *Affect regulation, mentalization, and the development of the self*. Routledge.

13. Good, G. E., & Brooks, G. R. (Eds.). (2005). *The new handbook of psychotherapy and counseling with men*. Jossey-Bass.

14. Gottman, J. M., & Levenson, R. W. (1992). Marital processes predictive of later dissolution: Behavior, physiology, and health. *Journal of Personality and Social Psychology, 63*(2), 221-233.

15. Grant, B. F., Chou, S. P., Goldstein, R. B., Huang, B., Stinson, F. S., Saha, T. D., Smith, S. M., Dawson, D. A., Pulay, A. J., Pickering, R. P., & Ruan, W. J. (2008). Prevalence, correlates, disability, and comorbidity of DSM-IV borderline personality disorder: Results from the Wave 2 National Epidemiologic Survey on Alcohol and Related Conditions. *Journal of Clinical Psychiatry, 69*(4), 533-545.

16. Hammer, J. H., & Vogel, D. L. (2010). Men's help seeking for depression: The efficacy of a male-sensitive brochure about counseling. *The Counseling Psychologist, 38*(2), 296-313.

17. Hazan, C., & Shaver, P. (1987). Romantic love conceptualized as an attachment process. *Journal of Personality and Social Psychology, 52*(3), 511-524.

18. Johnson, S. M. (2019). *Attachment in psychotherapy*. Guilford Publications.

19. Kreisman, J. J., & Straus, H. (2021). *Sometimes I act crazy: Living with borderline personality disorder*. Wiley.

20. Levant, R. F., & Pollack, W. S. (Eds.). (2003). *A new psychology of men*. Basic Books.

21. Levy, K. N., Meehan, K. B., Weber, M., Reynoso, J., & Clarkin, J. F. (2005). Attachment and borderline personality disorder: Implications for psychotherapy. *Psychopathology, 38*(2), 64-74.

22. Linehan, M. M. (2015). *DBT skills training manual* (2nd ed.). Guilford Press.

23. Linehan, M. M. (2020). *Building a life worth living: A memoir*. Random House.

24. Mahalik, J. R., Good, G. E., & Englar-Carlson, M. (2003). Masculinity scripts, presenting concerns, and help seeking: Implications for practice and training. *Professional Psychology: Research and Practice, 34*(2), 123-131.

25. Main, M., & Solomon, J. (1986). Discovery of an insecure-disorganized/disoriented attachment pattern. In T. B. Brazelton & M. W. Yogman (Eds.), *Affective development in infancy* (pp. 95-124). Ablex Publishing.

26. Manning, S. Y. (2011). *Loving someone with borderline personality disorder: How to keep out-of-control emotions from destroying your relationship*. Guilford Press

27. Mason, P. T., & Kreger, R. (2020). *Stop walking on eggshells: Taking your life back when someone you care*

about has borderline personality disorder (3rd ed.). New Harbinger Publications.

28. Nowinski, J. (2014). *Hard to love: Understanding and overcoming male borderline personality disorder.* Central Recovery Press.

29. O'Neil, J. M. (2008). Summarizing 25 years of research on men's gender role conflict using the Gender Role Conflict Scale: New research paradigms and clinical implications. *The Counseling Psychologist, 36(3),* 358-445.

30. Pistole, M. C. (1989). Attachment in adult romantic relationships: Style of conflict resolution and relationship satisfaction. *Journal of Social and Personal Relationships, 6(4),* 505-510.

31. Real, T. (1997). *I don't want to talk about it: Overcoming the secret legacy of male depression.* Scribner.

32. Reiland, R. (2018). *Get me out of here: My recovery from borderline personality disorder.* Hazelden Publishing.

33. Robertson, J. M., & Fitzgerald, L. F. (1992). Overcoming the masculine mystique: Preferences for alternative forms of assistance among men who avoid counseling. *Journal of Counseling Psychology, 39(2),* 240-246.

34. Roth, K., & Friedman, F. B. (2003). *Surviving a borderline parent: How to heal your childhood wounds and build trust, boundaries, and self-esteem.* New Harbinger Publications.

35. Santangelo, P., Bohus, M., & Ebner-Priemer, U. W. (2014). Ecological momentary assessment in borderline personality disorder: A review of recent findings and methodological challenges. *Journal of Personality Disorders, 28(4),* 555-576.

36. Simpson, J. A., & Rholes, W. S. (Eds.). (2015). *Attachment theory and research: New directions and emerging themes.* Guilford Press.

37. Skodol, A. E., Gunderson, J. G., Shea, M. T., McGlashan, T. H., Morey, L. C., Sanislow, C. A., Bender, D. S., Grilo, C. M., Zanarini, M. C., Yen, S., Pagano, M. E., & Stout, R. L. (2005). The Collaborative Longitudinal Personality Disorders Study (CLPS): Overview and implications. *Journal of Personality Disorders, 19*(5), 487-504.

38. Van Gelder, K. (2010). *The Buddha and the borderline: My recovery from borderline personality disorder through dialectical behavior therapy, Buddhism, and online dating.* New Harbinger Publications.

39. Zanarini, M. C., Frankenburg, F. R., Reich, D. B., & Fitzmaurice, G. (2012). Attainment and stability of sustained symptomatic remission and recovery among patients with borderline personality disorder and axis II comparison subjects: A 16-year prospective follow-up study. *American Journal of Psychiatry, 169*(5), 476-483.

www.ingramcontent.com/pod-product-compliance
Lightning Source LLC
Chambersburg PA
CBHW071724090426
42738CB00009B/1872